Intermitte
16/8 for Women

Achieve Hormone Harmony to Lose Weight Fast Without Losing Your Mind

Mag. Stephan Lederer, BSc, MSc

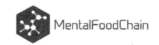

www.mentalfoodchain.com

This book is designed as an informational resource only. The information contained in this book should in no way be considered a substitute for the advice of a qualified physician, who should always be consulted before beginning any new diet, workout, or other health programs. Every effort has been made to ensure the accuracy of the information contained in this book at the time of publication. The author expressly disclaims responsibility for any adverse effects resulting from the use or application of the information contained in this book.

Some links in this eBook are affiliate links. Therefore, I may receive a tiny commission without incurring additional costs. In any case, the products must meet my high standards. Consequently, I recommend them because they are helpful, not because of the small commissions.

*Nobody should need a Ph.D. to balance hor-
mones naturally.*

Contents

Foreword

Have you ever felt misled by the contradictory dietary advice out there?

Are you looking for the first guide that understands your body?

If so, you've come to the right place!

This guide aims to create awareness of how your lifestyle and diet affect your body.

I believe health and well-being are about more than following dietary guidelines without transparent cause-and-effect relationships.

Once you understand the few crucial processes in your body, you can leverage them to optimize your health.

We have all put our trust in healthcare professionals. But who makes sure they stay on top of the latest research?

The fact is that for many people, the learning ends when they graduate. Moreover, it takes decades for scientific findings to find their way into textbooks.

For this reason, over 400 up-to-date studies, carefully researched, form the basis on which this guide, written in simple terms, is built.

Consequently, for the first time, hormones take the place of calorie values and are the focus of all considerations in this book.

Thanks to science, we now know that they significantly regulate our well-being, body weight, and life expectancy.

Unfortunately, the essentiality of hormones is still significantly underrepresented in health and diet advice. One of the primary reasons is that many hormones were not even known or measurable some years ago.

They are crucial to understanding how diet and lifestyle affect the body.

Understanding essential hormones can unleash the fat-burning and self-healing powers of the human body.

And the most effective way to do so is with intermittent fasting.

Admittedly, it takes a particular natural curiosity to question conventional wisdom about diet, which powerful industries and their campaigns have significantly influenced for decades.

If you didn't already have some doubts that more exercise and less calorie intake can be the panacea to all problems, you probably wouldn't have gotten as far as this paragraph.

An essential starting point of this book is the biological principle of homeostasis. Our bodies do not function like scales. Instead, they aim to maintain equilibriums for most vital functions.

Our western way of eating has nevertheless managed over decades to bring many hormones out of balance insidiously.

Therefore, in the information age, it is time to take our health back into our own hands.

For this reason, I would like to help you not be educated by marketing campaigns and dietary guidelines that powerful industrial lobbies' have fundamentally influenced anymore.

Small, little-known insights can make significant differences.

This guide gives you step-by-step information to help you build awareness of how your body works and reacts.

For this reason, I based it on a clear content structure that will allow you to optimize your health effortlessly.

The way to take your well-being back into your own hands with the least effort is through three simple sections:

I. **Hormones:** Get to know your hormones.

II. **Fasting:** Understand the effects of intermittent fasting on the female body.

III. **Lifestyle:** Develop a lifestyle that suits your daily routine and brings you happiness.

The health, fitness, and food industry's idea that you must constantly suffer and struggle to lose excess body fat and be healthy is simply wrong.

This guide empowers you to get into the shape you deserve without spending all your spare time in the gym and kitchen, following complicated recipes and portioning them.

Real Added Value for Women

Congratulations, you have purchased the first intermittent fasting book that understands your hormones and other crucial characteristics of your body and doesn't put you behind the stove for hours!

Unlike other books, I don't market a mere fad diet but rather educate you in easy-to-understand terms about crucial processes in your body.

When you understand how to regulate your hormones with intermittent fasting properly, you will achieve lasting results without starving or putting your health at risk!

Be clear about one thing:

Diets that don't fit into your daily routine, require complicated recipes and sinfully expensive foods, and severely restrict caloric intake end up in yo-yo dieting.[1]

Not to mention, such added stress in your daily work routine not only counteracts weight loss but also causes you to lose motivation sooner rather than later.

After reading this book, you'll know how to fast consistently, confidently, and safely without upsetting your hormones and menstrual cycle or wasting time and money.

Whether you're looking for more energy and focus at work, want to lose 30 pounds, fit into your old pants, or feel good about yourself: With this science-backed knowledge, it's possible with less effort than you might think.

Plus, this guide saves you all the hot air that other books on intermittent fasting are filled with, such as:

- 600 trendy exotic recipes that will prevent you from losing weight, give you hours in the kitchen, cravings, fatigue, and mood swings

- Guilt when you spend your spare time with family and friends instead of at the gym

- The hassle of counting calories, portioning, and tracking all your meals

- Taking highly processed diet foods and potentially harmful pharmaceutical products that throw your hormones out of balance

- Enumerating countless extreme fasting methods that won't fit your daily routine or produce lasting results

- Historical stories about diets that have nothing in common with intermittent fasting

- Myths about the metabolism, which lack any scientific evidence

Instead, you get a guide in simple words that takes you by the hand and leads to your health targets through tiny changes:

- How to optimize your hormone balance for fat loss

- How to control cravings without medication

- When and why the female body can react sensitively to dietary changes

- How to fast correctly and safely without upsetting your cycle

- How to eat right in every phase of the female cycle

- How to reduce premenstrual syndrome symptoms naturally with intermittent fasting

- What prevents you from losing weight with intermittent fasting and how to break through a weight-loss plateau

- What clean and dirty fasting is, and which variant offers the best results

- The role of exercise in weight loss and when you should or should not do it

- Whether intermittent fasting is safe and makes sense before, after, and during pregnancy

- Which beginner's mistakes to avoid not ruin results or lose motivation when starting with intermittent fasting

Even though this book is based on hundreds of studies, intermittent fasting is not rocket science.

In the age of abundance, intermittent fasting is the most straightforward and effective approach to balancing crucial hormones naturally.

Intermittent fasting 16/8 is so simple that it can get by with just one rule. And even to follow it, you don't have to do anything. All you have to do is skip one meal.

Unlike conventional diets, calorie restriction is not essential to intermittent fasting.

Intermittent fasting is not denying food intake. Instead, it is delaying it to a dedicated eating period.

Hence, you don't have to restrict or starve yourself.

However, studies show that people who eat fewer meals daily subconsciously consume less energy than others.[2]

By naturally balancing feasting and fasting, your hormone balance is set back to burn fat.

Let's take a detailed look at how this works.

PART I: HORMONES

Blood Sugar and Weight Loss

They regulate metabolism, appetite, and fat storage. Yet, in the conventional fitness industry, hormones don't even play a minor role in weight loss.

That anyone who puts too many pounds on the scale should eat less and exercise more is still the general view on weight loss today.

But are we just too lazy? After all, women, in particular, have never before been as ambitious to live a healthy life.

Do we move too little on average today to be able to lose weight, as some family doctors want us to tell?

Do billions of people voluntarily decide to overeat every day?

Whoever answers these questions with yes, has probably done the math without critical hormones.

The Key Role of Hormones

Hormones are chemical messengers that can provide critical signals to regulate hunger, satiety, thirst, body temperature, or even body weight.[3]

With the help of a control center in the brain, the hypothalamus, hormone balance is vital to keep bodily functions in a healthy equilibrium.

This biological principle of homeostasis also applies to essential metabolic processes. Once your hormones are out of whack, losing weight is hard.

Hormones decide whether you store energy or mobilize it, whether you are hungry or full, and how fat deposits are distributed around the body.

It's not due to a mere lack of willpower that more than 75% of adults in the US are already overweight or obese.[4]

If your hormonal course is set incorrectly, no matter how much you restrain yourself from eating or how often you exercise weekly, you won't lose weight successfully.

That's why world-renowned endocrinologist Dr. Robert Lustig concludes that the current obesity pandemic is due to a hormonal imbalance, not a caloric one.

The hormonal system plays the primary role in the development of obesity, even though cultural changes of the last half-century initiated it.[5]

And this Western lifestyle has long ceased to be a purely American problem but rather a global one.

Why Diets Fail

Hormones are the missing piece of the puzzle as to why eating less and exercising more over the past several decades has not inevitably led to success.

Because of the varying impact of foods on hormone balance, a calorie is not always a calorie. A study from Great Britain shows that the simplified calorie counting approach does not work.

In this study, 99.5% of 99,791 overweight women and 76,704 overweight men were unable to lose weight successfully through a classic calorie deficit.[6]

Our body is not a combustion engine that runs equally well on any fuel source, no matter how dirty. Instead, its life expectancy depends on the quality of food.

Because it is not a closed system, the laws of thermodynamics do not apply to our bodies.

Instead, the biological principle of homeostasis applies since the human body is an open, dynamic system. And our hormones play a crucial role in signaling.

So why is calorie counting still the standard of the fitness industry?

Because this allows industrially produced foods such as protein bars or vegan butter to sell first-class. Moreover, this fake food is shelf-stable almost forever.

The ongoing obesity pandemic is a composition of increasingly stressful lives and the industrialization of food.

Eating less and exercising more is not a recipe for fixing this toxic lifestyle. You may lose weight with it in the short term, but whether it is body fat that you are losing is determined by your hormones.

A study conducted on participants in the weight-loss TV series The Biggest Loser shows that people cannot lose weight sustainably with calorie reduction and exercise if hormones are left out of the equation.

Thus, the participants who lost the most weight through calorie restriction still suffered from an overwhelmingly reduced basal metabolic rate six years later.[7]

Because of this yo-yo effect, conventional dieting does not work. The reason is the hormones involved in weight loss, first and foremost our fat-storage hormone.

When small meals constantly stimulate insulin, you can't break down body fat, and the body burns lean mass instead. Let's have a look at how this works.

Storage Hormone Insulin

The most important hormone when it comes to losing weight is insulin. Most people have heard of insulin and immediately associate it with diabetes.

That's because regulating blood sugar levels is one of this messenger's essential tasks. Since excess sugar molecules in the blood are harmful, the body strives to control the amount of sugar (glucose) in the blood.

The fastest way to rid the blood of glucose is to transport it into the cells to be used as energy or stored as fat.

And insulin is responsible for precisely regulating the amount of glucose in the blood.

Accordingly, insulin plays an essential role in supplying energy to cells. On the other hand, it is also our primary storage hormone.

Finally, insulin also signals fat cells to take up excess energy that cannot be used at the moment.

In addition, the fat-storage hormone has a so-called antilipolytic effect.[8]

That means that it prevents the breakdown of fat by enzymes (lipolysis) and promotes fat storage.[9]

In short, high insulin levels prevent fat burning.

Since insulin's role is to regulate blood glucose, it is only legitimate that its presence blocks the drawing of additional energy from fat stores.

Accordingly, when you supply an adequate amount of glucose by eating carbohydrates, insulin does a first-rate job of consuming that energy.

However, if too much glucose enters the bloodstream due to high carbohydrate consumption, insulin ensures that the excess energy is stored in fat cells.[10]

The most effective way to lower insulin levels is to abstain from food intake for some time strictly.

Accordingly, 107 overweight young women study shows that intermittent fasting can significantly reduce insulin levels and resistance.[11]

Insulin resistance is a protective mechanism of the body against excessive insulin levels, which could otherwise be life-threatening. As a result, cells are less sensitive to insulin.

It develops when the body constantly produces insulin, for example, when people eat carbohydrates around the clock.

Insulin resistance is a metabolic condition and precursor to type 2 diabetes and metabolic syndrome.[12]

It is a vicious cycle, as the body has to secrete more and more insulin to maintain essential functions.

The seriousness with which Western lifestyles disrupt insulin balance is demonstrated by the fact that in 2016, over 50% of the US population already had at least one pre-diabetes condition.[13]

Antagonist Glucagon

In the context of blood glucose, there exists another player besides insulin that you need to get to know. In short, glucagon is the antagonist of insulin.

While insulin is released by increasing blood sugar, your body releases glucagon when the blood sugar gets too low.

Therefore, glucagon pursues the same goal as insulin: it wants to keep blood sugar in balance. Both hormones thus target what is known as blood glucose homeostasis.

Consequently, it is hardly surprising that glucagon is also produced in the pancreas. In contrast to insulin, secretion occurs through alpha instead of beta cells.

Unlike insulin, which lowers a high blood glucose level, glucagon raises low blood glucose.[14]

For this purpose, two mechanisms exist in the body:

- On the one hand, glucagon can stimulate the liver to break down glucose from carbohydrate stores (glycogen).

- On the other hand, glucagon can signal fat cells to release stored fat.

In summary, glucagon is a hormone that mobilizes stored energy and stimulates sugar and fat burning. On the other hand, its counterpart, insulin, stores energy and blocks fat burning.

Proper fasting sets the hormonal course for weight loss.

A study conducted at Harvard Medical School supports this fact. While the insulin levels of the participating subjects dropped, glucagon levels doubled on the third day of fasting and slowly declined over the following six weeks, always remaining above baseline.[15]

Stress Hormone Cortisol

Psychological stress is an essential part of our Western lifestyle. That is why stress has long ceased to play a minor role in weight loss.

The adrenal glands secrete cortisol in response to stress. Accordingly, cortisol is considered an essential stress hormone.

Cortisol is crucial to prepare the body for fight or flight.

Therefore, the standard repertoire of physiological responses to stressful situations that cortisol initiates is called the fight-or-flight response.

After cortisol is released, it immediately increases blood sugar (glucose). For this reason, studies show that stress can trigger cravings for sweets.[16]

The mobilized energy aims at strengthening muscles and eventually being able to escape and survive.[17]

This response to acute stress was essential for survival during evolution. However, in chronic stress, cortisol can have harmful effects.

Due to psychological stress, blood glucose levels can remain high for months, stimulating insulin release. Accordingly, persistently high cortisol levels lead to significantly elevated insulin levels.[18]

And the storage hormone is known to be a primary contributor to obesity. Thus, psychological stress increases body mass index and abdominal fat over time.[19]

In addition, researchers have found that an enzyme that can reactivate inactive cortisol (cortisone) is elevated in the abdominal fat of obese individuals.[20]

As a result, these individuals show increased body mass index (BMI), obesity around the middle, and associated disease risks.[21]

To manage cortisol levels, you must focus on minimizing stress responses, which is not always easy in everyday life.

Ultimately, you cannot avoid many psychological stressors.

For this reason, mindfulness-based stress reduction techniques such as yoga or meditation have gained immense popularity in recent years.

How Eating Can Make You Sick

Although humans in modern societies typically eat at least three times a day, they evolved in an environment where food was relatively scarce.

As a result, we developed numerous adaptations that enable us to function at a high level, both physically and mentally, in a food-deprived state.[22]

Therefore, eating foods in these modern dietary patterns often leads to metabolic disease.

When we eat carbohydrates and proteins, the pancreas secretes insulin.

As the primary storage hormone, insulin ensures that supplied energy is stored for later use.

This natural mechanism has allowed humanity to survive famines.

The liver is the essential organ for storing and distributing energy in the body. It stores excess blood sugar preferentially as glycogen in the liver and partially in skeletal muscle.

This compound of three to four parts water and one part glucose can be quickly converted into energy by the liver.

However, glycogen stores are limited. On average, a woman can store about 1900 kcal of energy as glycogen. That's about a day's worth of fuel.

In contrast, body fat is an unlimited storage medium.

When glycogen stores in the liver are full, it initiates *de novo lipogenesis*.

This process converts excess glucose into triglycerides and distributes them throughout the body as follows:

- Under the skin (subcutaneous fat)
- In the liver (fatty liver)
- In other organs (visceral fat)

The exciting thing is that this way, saturated fat enters the blood. However, this fat is not derived from dietary fats but from carbohydrates.

Accordingly, recent studies show that saturated fats from food reduce heart disease while carbohydrates increase it.[23]

Because the human body has glycogen stores for short-term and body fat for long-term energy reserves, it is designed for a balance of feasting and fasting.

You may have heard that we lose weight mainly while sleeping. Since insulin levels decrease during sleep, insulin is less able to prevent weight loss.

Without food intake, insulin levels drop, allowing glycogen and body fat to be converted back into energy and used.

However, we have entirely suppressed that we can and should go more than eight hours without constant snacking.

Advertising campaigns have drilled absurd notions into us for decades, such as that we need six meals a day to lose weight.

Therefore, the average person rarely taps into body fat for energy because they constantly eat and produce insulin.

Because of the imbalance between eating and fasting, we now have excessively high insulin levels, which are the perfect recipe for obesity and modern diseases.

The characteristics of metabolic syndrome explain why too much insulin in the body threatens health.

These are composed of the following contemporary severe health risks:[24]

- High blood sugar (due to insulin resistance)
- Elevated blood lipid levels (triglycerides)
- High blood pressure (hypertension)
- Low HDL levels (high-density lipoprotein, good cholesterol)
- Obesity (adiposity)

All of these factors contribute significantly to those modern and chronic diseases that plague us most today:[25,26,27,28]

- Strokes, heart attacks, and other cardiovascular diseases
- Type 2 diabetes
- Cancer
- Alzheimer's disease
- Parkinson's disease

In 1988, Dr. Gerald Reaven of Stanford University received one of the highest honors in diabetes research for making an exciting discovery.[29]

Not only do the characteristics of metabolic syndrome, but also modern diseases have the same root cause: *Hyperinsulinemia*.[30]

These excessively high insulin levels and the resulting insulin resistance are major factors in the mortality rates of our modern society.

In short, for seven of the ten leading death causes in Western countries, high insulin levels facilitated by diet and lifestyle are significant factors.[31]

In addition, we now also know that people who have these metabolic syndrome risk factors are significantly more vulnerable to coronavirus and die.[32]

In contrast, fewer meals per day can counteract the development of diseases and improve a wide range of age-related conditions, including diabetes, cardiovascular diseases, cancer, Alzheimer's, and Parkinson's disease.[33]

Hunger and Satiety

As the control center for appetite, the hypothalamus in the brain also coordinates eating behavior.[34]

Hunger and satiety hormones provide the brain with information about how much energy you have already consumed and how much you still need.

The goal is energy homeostasis: Balancing energy production (metabolism) and energy consumption in cells.[35]

This chapter reviews the major hormones involved in balancing hunger and satiety.

In addition to the chemical messengers on this list, other hormones and neurotransmitters can influence appetite regulation.

However, the following hormones are the best researched to understand how they affect our food intake.

In addition, sufficient research exists regarding these six hunger and satiety hormones to infer the influence of modern lifestyle factors on hormone balance.

For this reason, we can also derive how we can naturally regulate these hormones.

First among them is the essential initiator of appetite.

Hunger Hormone Ghrelin

Ghrelin is better known as the hunger hormone. And for a good reason. Ultimately, ghrelin is the only neurotransmitter outside the central nervous system that triggers appetite.[36]

The body releases ghrelin in response to an empty stomach to tell you to eat again shortly.[37]

Additionally, the reward center in your brain is stimulated to make food more attractive to you.[38]

After a meal, on the other hand, ghrelin levels are low. When the stomach is full, there is no longer a need for food intake.

A healthy ghrelin level correlates negatively with body fat, i.e., it is higher in lean individuals and lowers in obese individuals.[39]

However, in obese people, ghrelin levels do not always decrease as they should after a meal. Because they continue to feel hungry, these people risk overeating.[40]

Consequently, an imbalance in ghrelin secretion can lead to weight gain. Conversely, ghrelin balance must function properly to lose weight successfully.

Satiety Hormone Leptin

Leptin is the counterpart of the hunger hormone ghrelin. Accordingly, it is also known as the satiety hormone.

Unlike ghrelin, leptin has to do directly with body fat. It is the fat cells themselves that produce the hormone.

When you eat and your fat cells determine that you've put in enough energy, they release leptin, which signals the brain to stop eating.

If your leptin levels are low, on the other hand, your brain receives the message that fat stores are empty, which in turn triggers hunger.[41]

Consequently, leptin is responsible for regulating the body's total amount of stored energy. Hence, leptin levels correlate positively with your body fat.[42]

When the signaling to regulate body fat stops working correctly, it is called leptin resistance.

When the body is constantly flooded with high amounts of leptin, it becomes less responsive to the hormonal signal over time. Therefore, leptin sensitivity decreases.

In short, with leptin resistance, your brain takes longer to recognize that you're already full.

The result can be overeating, weight gain, obesity, and other metabolic disorders.[43]

Leptin resistance is associated with chronic inflammation, obesity, cardiovascular disease, insulin resistance, and type 2 diabetes.[44]

Researchers hypothesize that excessive levels of the storage hormone insulin, which is also instrumental in weight gain, cause leptin resistance.[45]

The more you eat those foods that stimulate insulin secretion, the worse leptin or insulin resistance can become.

In addition to the well-known satiety hormone leptin, three other hormones inhibit appetite and have already been researched well. They are all mainly produced in your intestine.

In addition, research is aware of an extraordinarily exciting hormone that triggers hunger in the brain. Since it closely interacts with the primary hunger and satiety hormones, let's look at the neurotransmitter in detail.

Neuropeptide Y

With neuropeptide Y (NPY), we move into the central nervous system. There it is the most abundant peptide.

NPY is primarily found in the hypothalamus and is a hormone and a neurotransmitter. Moreover, NPY is considered the most potent appetite-stimulating compound in the human body.

Every other hunger or satiety hormone regulates food intake by acting on NPY in the hypothalamus. While leptin suppresses NPY activity, ghrelin stimulates it.[46]

Accordingly, elevated NPY increases food cravings, predominantly carbohydrates.[47]

For this reason, like ghrelin, we can refer to it as a hunger hormone.

In addition to hunger, NPY stimulates fat storage and weight gain via the central nervous system while decreasing sex drive, locomotion, energy expenditure, and body temperature.[48]

Moreover, stress increases NPY levels in fat cells, contributing to abdominal fat storage.[49]

However, elevated NPY levels make sense as a stress response because NPY has stress-reducing, anxiety-relieving, and neuroprotective properties, according to researchers at the University of Graz, Austria.[50]

You may have also heard that researchers have found that many living things can live at least 33% longer if they eat less.[51]

Because NPY acts as the primary hunger signal in this context, researchers suspect it plays an essential role in extending lifespan.[52]

Peptide YY

Like NPY, peptide YY (PYY) is a crucial brain-gut peptide. Therefore, the actions of both peptides are closely related to appetite regulation and the development of obesity.[53]

PYY is produced in the intestine after eating. Here, the amount secreted is proportional to the fat ingested with food.[54]

It enters the hypothalamus in the brain via the bloodstream, reducing appetite.[55]

Hence, it is a satiety hormone.

According to studies, individuals with obesity exhibited attenuated peptide YY responses after eating, leading to uncontrolled overeating.[56]

Therefore, adequate PYY levels are essential in reducing increased food intake, especially after extensive exercise.[57]

In addition, researchers at Oxford have found that obese individuals do not already have high fasting PYY levels, but chronic overeating elevates them.

According to the researchers, this suggests a protective mechanism against excessive food intake and other satiety hormones.[58]

Glucagon-Like Peptide-1

The next satiety hormone, glucagon-like peptide-1 (GLP-1), is secreted along with PYY in the gut in response to nutrient intake.

Its main functions are to keep blood glucose levels stable and produce a feeling of satiety.[59]

This hormone could also help weight loss and reduce body mass index (BMI) or waist circumference in overweight adults.[60]

Moreover, researchers explain the reduced hunger and increased satiety after gastric bypass surgery by an increased GLP-1 response to food intake.[61]

The beneficial effects of GLP-1 make this hormone an exciting candidate for treating obesity, diabetes, and neurodegenerative diseases.[62]

Research suggests that people with obesity may experience problems with GLP-1 signaling.[63]

As with the other appetite hormones, this suggests a possible type of GLP-1 resistance. This decreasing GLP-1 sensitivity may also explain the elevated fasted plasma GLP-1 levels in obese children and adults.[64]

Cholecystokinin

The last in our series of satiety hormones is cholecystokinin (CCK). Also, cells in the gut produce CCK in response to a meal.

CCK is the first gut hormone known to affect appetite.[65] It is closely related to the primary satiety hormone leptin.

On the one hand, CCK promotes leptin secretion.[66] On the other hand, leptin enhances CCK-induced satiety.[67]

An elevated CCK level can be detected in the human body approximately 15 minutes after eating.[68]

In addition to satiety, cholecystokinin also plays an essential role in the following processes in the body:[69]

- Inhibition of gastric acid secretion and release of digestive enzymes

- Contraction of the gallbladder and regulation of bile acid

- Regulation of gastric emptying

- Energy production, protein synthesis, and cell growth

Our bodies produce CCK when we consume protein or fat.[70]

As a result, food intake and, in particular, our cravings for sugar and carbohydrates are reduced.[71]

Recent research suggests that obese people develop a type of CCK resistance. Reduced sensitivity to the hormone makes them more likely to overeat, which may contribute to the progression of CCK resistance.[72]

Sexuality and Fertility

Many people think that the sex hormones estrogen and testosterone are mortal enemies, always fighting a bitter hormone war.

Some women even fear that weight lifting and eating meat could cause increased testosterone levels and result in an overly masculine appearance.

On the other hand, few people know that testosterone also performs essential tasks in the female body. For example, testosterone is instrumental in estrogen production, which is why a deficiency also affects it.

Estrogen

Estrogen is the primary sex hormone in women. Nevertheless, estrogen is also naturally present in male bodies, but not in such high amounts.

In addition to its primary function in female reproduction and sex drive in both sexes, the hormone also plays a role in fat distribution.

However, the reduction of estrogen levels does not lead to weight loss. Due to this fact, menopausal women tend to gain abdominal fat despite lower estrogen levels.[73]

For this reason, estrogen levels are a sensitive issue. Hence, they must be regulated carefully: Neither too high nor too low will help you lose weight.

However, in addition to hormonal changes throughout the life cycle, lifestyle factors can keep estrogen levels at the right level, as we will learn shortly.

Testosterone

Testosterone occurs as a chemical messenger in both men and women.

Although most people associate testosterone exclusively with men, women also produce testosterone.

Women produce most of their testosterone in the ovaries.

The rest is produced in body fat and skin tissue in response to two steroid hormones:

- *Dehydroepiandrosterone (DHEA)* from the adrenal glands
- *Androstenedione* from the ovaries

Estrogen is also produced there. And the production of the female sex hormone requires testosterone.

Consequently, a certain hormonal balance of testosterone and estrogen is essential for both men and women, even if it does not occur to the same extent in the different sexes.

A healthy testosterone level contributes significantly to the following aspects of the human body:[74]

- mood
- libido
- muscle mass
- bone density
- body fat distribution

Accordingly, testosterone is a hormone that also plays an essential role in weight loss. It is therefore also referred to as a fat-reducing hormone.[75]

However, compared to women, the consequences of impaired testosterone balance can be more extreme for men.

Therefore, researchers even conclude that an increase in the hormone in men directly results in the loss of abdominal fat.[76]

If testosterone levels drop significantly in men, the balance to estrogen is compromised. As a result, fatty tissue may grow on the chest.[77]

Another hormone in the blood regulates the presence of estrogen and testosterone.

Called sex hormone-binding globulin (SHBG), it binds the sex hormones in the blood, keeping them in balance.

After our conventional high-carbohydrate Western diet drives up insulin levels, the body can no longer secrete enough SHBG.[78]

You gain body fat more easily when testosterone and estrogen balance is out of whack.

That's another reason to practice intermittent fasting – the most effective method to lower insulin levels.

Menstrual Cycle

Before diving into how intermittent fasting can affect your fertility hormones and the female body, it's first essential to understand how the menstrual cycle works.

Each cycle is individual. Understanding how your menstrual cycle works is the first important step in optimizing hormone balance and health.

Accordingly, a regular female cycle duration can range from 26 to 35 days.[79]

Each menstrual cycle has two main phases: The follicular and luteal phases. In this context, ovulation initiates the turning point between these main phases.

This exemplary cycle spans an average duration of 28 days.[80]

Follicular Phase (Menstrual Cycle Day 1-13)

The follicular phase begins on the first day of your period and continues until ovulation. Again, this phase can be divided into two subphases: The menstrual and proliferation phases.

Menstrual Phase (Menstrual Cycle Day 1-4)

At the beginning of this phase, levels of the hormones estrogenic and progesterone are low.[81]

Due to low progesterone levels, we shed the functional layer of the endometrium.

The menstrual phase may last 3-7 days.

Proliferation Phase (Menstrual Cycle Day 5-13)

During the proliferation phase, follicle-stimulating hormone (FSH) is stimulated to mature the follicles in the ovaries that contain the eggs.

Estrogen levels increase and peak at ovulation.[82]

During this process, the influence of the sex hormone causes the uterine lining to build up.

Ovulation (Menstrual Cycle Day 14)

The ovulation initiates the turn between the follicular and luteal phases.

Accordingly, it occurs around the middle of the cycle. Ovulation is characterized by a significant increase in FSH and luteinizing hormone (LH), while estrogen levels begin to drop briefly.[83]

For this reason, the egg is released from the ovaries. Therefore, ovulation is the right time for pregnancy.

However, if fertilization of the egg does not occur within 24 hours, the egg dies.

Luteal Phase (Menstrual Cycle Day 15-28)

After ovulation, the luteal phase begins, characterized by decreased FSH and LH.

The corpus luteum develops from the follicle (shell of the egg). It produces the hormone progesterone under the influence of LH.

Therefore, during the luteal phase, progesterone levels begin to rise sharply. Estrogen levels also slowly increase again.[84]

If no fertilized egg has nested in the endometrium, the corpus luteum regresses, and the corpus luteum hormone progesterone decreases.

Also, estrogen falls again at the end of the luteal phase, stimulating the follicular phase and thus a new cycle.

Now that we know about all the essential hormones that can affect body fat, appetite, and well-being, the second central part of the book deals with how intermittent fasting affects the female body.

In it, you'll learn why intermittent fasting can effort-lessly maximize a woman's health when practiced correctly.

PART II: FASTING

What Is Fasting?

Fasting means not eating any food for a certain period.

Since water cannot significantly affect the health effects of fasting, only religiously motivated fasting sometimes restricts fluid intake.

However, in therapeutic and intermittent fasting, fluid intake is essential. However, do not consume liquid foods (smoothies, juices, etc.) or fluids that significantly stimulate insulin secretion during periods of fasting.

You can find out precisely what you can drink during intermittent fasting in my detailed guide:

What Can You Drink During Intermittent Fasting – the Science of Fasting Explained (affiliate link).

In contrast, food is strictly prohibited during the fasting period. We will look at why energy intake during the fasting window affects weight loss and health benefits shortly.

As a traditional health practice, fasting has been used not only for weight loss but also for the following purposes:

- Improved mental focus
- Prevention of dementia
- Prevention of insulin resistance
- Slowing down the aging process

This ancient healing tradition's roots lie primarily in autophagy – an intracellular recycling process science is currently unraveling.

In addition, fasting has been used in various spiritual methods. That fasting can help you suppress emotional urges, think clearly, and thus make better decisions might be a primary reason.

Regardless of your spiritual beliefs, fasting can help you get closer to your true self and feel connected to the world around you.

While shorter duration fasting - so-called intermittent fasting - tends to be more common, some people also practice longer fasts.

Although widespread intermittent fasting methods usually have a fasting period of 12 to 24 hours, other types of fasting can last for several days.

History of Fasting

Fasting has been integral to virtually all cultures' traditional health and healing practices throughout recorded human history.

Moreover, this is true for virtually all regions and religions worldwide. Fasting has been used therapeutically since at least the 5th century BC.

Accordingly, Hippocrates, the Greek physician, and father of modern medicine, recommended abstinence from food and drink to patients who exhibited specific symptoms of illness.[85]

Similarly, other physicians reported a fasting instinct that may naturally lose appetite in patients in certain disease states.

Some physicians considered food administration unnecessary and possibly even harmful during such states, as fasting was considered an important natural part of the recovery process.

This view makes perfect sense based on the latest scientific findings.

Strict fasting induces autophagy. In short, this intracellular process activates the self-healing power of the human body.[86]

In the second half of the 19th century, an understanding of the physiological effects of fasting began to develop. The first organized fasting studies were conducted with animals and humans at this time.

In the 20th century, as more became known about the diet and nutritional needs of the human body, fasting methods became more sophisticated, and a wide range of approaches emerged.

Thus, fasting was used to treat and prevent disease in clinical settings.

These medical fasting methods were used primarily to treat chronic diseases and often lasted longer than a month. They allowed only the consumption of water or calorie-free tea.

In addition, these health-motivated fasting schedules included exercise and enemas.

Regrettably, the therapeutic use of fasting in medical and clinical settings has steadily declined after a high in the 1950s and 1960s.

The fact that eating less can bring various beneficial effects was probably difficult for the advancing consumer-centered society to comprehend.

It has regained immense popularity among health-conscious people since recent advances in biochemistry have made it possible to explain the processes behind the health benefits of fasting.

Intermittent Fasting

Intermittent fasting has become the most popular form due to its scientifically proven benefits.

It involves fasting within a certain period and eating only during the rest of the day or week.

There are various forms of intermittent fasting, but the most popular is fasting within a time window of around 16 hours.

For example, you eat exclusively between noon and 8 PM. This way, your body can fast for 16 hours out of 24 hours with an 8-hour eating window.

However, if you have special working hours, you can also skip dinner or lunch and be successful. This flexibility is one of the main practical advantages of intermittent fasting.

For this reason, there are hardly any limits to the possibilities of intermittent fasting.

Unlike other diet trends, intermittent fasting is about less, not more. As soon as you skip a meal, you're already practicing it. You don't need to buy expensive foods or gather an enormous collection of sophisticated recipes.

Prolonged Fasting

If the duration of fasting exceeds 48 hours, it is called prolonged fasting. More extended fasts can also have more intensive effects on the body.

Accordingly, they can deliver even more significant health benefits, such as:[87,88,89]

- Detoxification of the body
- Removal of pathogens
- Renewal of old and dysfunctional cell parts
- Reduction of bone and muscle atrophy
- Prevention of neurodegenerative diseases (e.g., Alzheimer's, Parkinson's)
- Prevention of cancer, insulin resistance, and type 2 diabetes
- Reversal of the aging process
- Extension of life span

However, a prolonged fast that lasts longer than 48 hours will probably reduce the digestive enzymes of the pancreas and intestines.

Therefore, resuming eating after a prolonged fast often requires more attention.

If we are used to eating continuously, the body needs some time to adapt to the fasting state. But this is logical, natural, and not particularly alarming.

Fasting gives the entire digestive tract time to recover, which it often lacks today.

Since the food industry educated us to eat the whole day continuously, our bodies frequently use metabolic energy to produce enzymes that can process the food.

Accordingly, you may know the feeling when all the energy and blood flow into the stomach and digestive tract. As a result, you can't think clearly after eating.

When we fast, the digestive enzymes are neither needed nor produced so that the body can supply the metabolic energy to other organs, such as the brain.[90]

For this reason, some people report sharpened focus, mental clarity, and increased productivity when fasting, which I can also confirm.

Top 10 Fasting Myths Debunked by Science

Many people panic about fasting, even though it is thoroughly natural.

Yes, there were times in human history when neither refrigerators nor supermarkets opened in winter.

As a logical consequence, humankind has always had to fast for many days. However, numerous myths have developed in the age of abundance that are difficult to get out of our heads.

Here are the top 10 myths about intermittent fasting and their clarification based on recent studies.

1. Frequent Small Meals Help You Lose Weight

Which is the better consumer: The one who eats 1-2 times a day and thus has time to prepare a high-quality meal or who eats every few hours and therefore relies on convenience foods?

Unfortunately, it's the latter. Advertising has educated us with adverse diet advice, including:

- Never skip a meal
- Snacks help you lose weight
- Many small meals boost metabolism
- You must eat six times a day to lose weight

This dietary advice gave rise to the notion that eating multiple meals increases the metabolic rate, causing the body to burn more calories overall.

Nonetheless, eating more often to lose weight is just as controversial as it sounds.

While a thermic effect of food does exist, requiring extra energy, mainly when proteins are digested, it cannot equalize the negative impact of snacking.

Accordingly, studies debunked this intermittent fasting myth since people who eat snacks eat more daily.[91]

Moreover, it is scientifically proven that snacks cannot help people lose weight.[92]

The reason for this is the influence of nutrition on our hormone balance. Ultimately, these messengers determine whether we gain or lose weight.

As we already know, insulin is the leading player in this context.[93]

Consequently, many meals ensure that insulin levels do not drop throughout the day. Thus, you make fat loss impossible and promote fat gain simultaneously.[94]

2. Fasting Puts Your Body in Starvation Mode

One of the oldest myths is that intermittent fasting causes the mysterious starvation mode. The term refers to the fear that the body shuts down the metabolism to save energy.

However, against starvation mode, we must distinguish between true fasting and conventional caloric restriction.

Intermittent fasting is not a conventional diet. Instead, it is an eating pattern that distinguishes between strict periods of feating and fasting.

It does not involve snacking and starving around the clock.

What people fear as starvation mode is nothing other than the yo-yo effect of conventional diets.

And what is the lowest common denominator of conventional diets? Calorie counting!

How conventional calorie reduction can permanently restrict the basal metabolic rate is best shown by a study conducted on participants of the weight-loss TV show The Biggest Loser.

It showed that the participants who lost the most weight through calorie restriction still significantly reduced basal metabolic rate six years later.[95]

Eating small meals frequently ensures that insulin levels barely drop throughout the day. Therefore, the body cannot break down stored fat for energy.[96]

However, unlike fasting, the body can access lean mass due to the lack of growth hormone protecting muscle.[97]

Consequently, daily caloric restriction decreases the basal metabolic rate. Ultimately, it must manage the restricted energy intake.

The longer the period of calorie restriction, the greater the adverse effects on metabolism. The result is better known as yo-yo dieting.

With intermittent fasting, on the other hand, the body does not go into energy-saving mode. After no energy is supplied, it must instead mobilize stored energy.

Why you don't collapse overtired during fasting will explain the hormonal system again.

3. Fasting Slows Down the Metabolism

The idea that many small meals could boost metabolism came from the notion that fewer meals per day should slow it down.

In contrast, scientists already debunked this sticky myth more than 50 years ago by showing that fasting instead boosts metabolism.[98]

Thus, nature has provided for difficult times. Would humankind still be today if our ancestors had immediately gone limp due to an unsuccessful hunt? Most likely not!

Due to the increased release of growth hormones, noradrenaline, and adrenaline, our ancestors could search for food longer when it was scarce.

Therefore, the hormonal system ensures that the basal metabolic rate remains high precisely when no energy is supplied.[99]

In addition, norepinephrine and epinephrine significantly help break down stored body fat.[100]

By mobilizing necessary energy while conserving muscle mass, species survival could be ensured.[101]

4. Intermittent Fasting Causes Muscle Loss

Contrary to popular myths, fasting does not cause muscles to atrophy.

The myth that fasting destroys muscle arose because protein can be broken down and used for energy when fasting for a sufficiently long time.

However, this is not muscle protein. Instead, the body focuses on defective proteins, for example, in the skin or intestinal mucosa.

This way, the body obtains amino acids that would otherwise be supplied with food.

Moreover, this intracellular recycling process of autophagy also protects against muscle breakdown.[102]

In fact, many of our metabolic pathways are designed to conserve muscle mass at all costs.

Also, the efficient fat-burning mechanism of fasting (ketosis) helps prevent muscle breakdown.[103]

Besides, the body releases so-called counter-regulatory hormones ensuring muscle mass remains intact during fasting.

One of these is the human growth hormone. During fasting, the release of growth hormone peaks to ensure you don't lose muscle mass.

For this reason, fasting is also a time-honored strategy for building muscle and is by no means a foreign concept in bodybuilder circles.

Since the natural release of growth hormones decreases with advancing age, intermittent fasting is increasingly crucial for muscle gain.

That intermittent fasting causes muscle loss is one of the most persistent myths

Yet intermittent fasting protects against muscle loss and bone mass from degeneration.[104]

Moreover, increased growth hormone release improves muscle recovery after exercise, organ health, and life expectancy.[105]

5. You Can Only Use Limited Protein per Meal

The idea that you need to eat protein every few hours and consume about 30 grams at every meal to build muscle is false.

Studies show that more frequent protein intake does not affect lean mass development.[106]

On the contrary, the total amount of protein consumed matters and not the number of meals it is distributed.

Likewise, a study on older women states that protein intake in large meals is more effective than spreading the same protein over small meals.[107]

Ultimately, the human body can absorb more significant amounts of protein at one time or store nutrients.

Because you can keep your insulin levels low longer, intermittent fasting is a method that can promote fat loss and muscle gain at the same time.

That's why 16/8 intermittent fasting is known as the *Lean Gains Method*. In bodybuilding, time-restricted eating has been used for decades to build muscle without gaining body fat precisely.

6. Fasting Induces Risky Blood Sugar Levels

In a world dominated by refined carbohydrates and sugar, it is an advantage that intermittent fasting can lower blood sugar.

However, myths evolved that the lower blood sugar induced by fasting could cause even fainting.

Nevertheless, according to research results, the blood sugar level remains stable even if you fast for a more extended period.[108]

Accordingly, several protective mechanisms are in line to guarantee healthy blood sugar.

Firstly, there are the body's carbohydrate stores in the liver and skeletal muscle mass. As long as this stored glycogen is present, the body uses it and converts it back into glucose.

Since full glycogen stores provide about your entire daily energy needs, they slowly become empty after 24 hours, at which point the body must start to tap into stored fat for energy.[109]

Finally, the so-called winter flab also has a function that has always ensured the survival of our species.

Fat energy sources can entirely supply all organs except the brain. However, it is not true that the brain is exclusively dependent on glucose, as we will learn shortly.

When carbohydrate stores are empty, gluconeo-genesis kicks in. This process describes the conversion of glycerol, lactate, and amino acids into glucose to ensure that blood glucose levels cannot become dangerously low.[110]

For this reason, essential carbohydrates do not exist, as we do not need them for survival.

Since gluconeogenesis establishes stable blood glucose, intermittent fasting helps eliminate mood swings. These originate from the blood sugar roller coaster that high carbohydrate diets cause.

Contrary to popular belief, it is not intermittent fasting, but the blood sugar crash following a food-induced blood sugar spike causing short-term hypo-glycemia.

7. The Brain Needs a Steady Glucose Supply

Also, about 75% of the brain's energy supply can be fed by fat energy yields because these so-called ketones can cross the blood-brain barrier.[111]

They are also the reason why people report increased mental clarity when fasting. Ketones are a kind of superfood for the brain.

Because the brain and other organs can use ketones more efficiently than carbohydrates, many people report improved mental clarity, mood, and reduced appetite in a state of ketosis.[112]

In addition, ketones have antioxidant and anti-inflammatory properties that help repair those cellular damages caused by refined carbohydrates and vegetable oils.[113,114]

The liver provides the remaining 25% of glucose needed to the brain through gluconeogenesis.

8. Fasting Causes Nutrient Deficiencies

That fasting could lead to a nutrient shortage is a legitimate concern. To examine this fear, we need to look at the spectrum of nutrients we might be lacking:

- Macronutrients
  - Fat
  - Protein
  - Carbohydrates
- Micronutrients
  - Vitamins
  - Minerals

People think primarily of vitamin deficiencies. However, it is almost impossible to cause a vitamin deficiency through intermittent fasting due to the eating period. However, optional vitamin supplementation is conceivable during long therapeutic fasting periods.

For example, doctors used a multivitamin in the fasting world record over 382 days. Although the researchers added potassium externally for a short period, they concluded it unnecessary.

Only after 200 days of fasting was an increased excretion of minerals detected. These were the electrolytes magnesium, sodium, potassium, and calcium.[115]

Against this background, bone broth is a popular aid in therapeutic fasting since it covers almost all essential minerals and vitamins.

That intermittent fasting causes nutrient deficiencies is among countless myths

However, with intermittent fasting, only the loss of sodium during the depletion of carbohydrate stores can cause side effects such as dizziness and headaches.

Nonetheless, drinking mineral water or homemade sole water can help.

Regarding macronutrients, it is apparent that we cannot develop a carbohydrate deficiency since there are no essential carbohydrates.

On the contrary, we must supply essential amino and fatty acids through food. However, the body's ambition to recycle fats and proteins increases as fasting progresses.

Accordingly, it excretes successively less through stool. But the body goes even further and recycles defective cell parts through autophagy, delivering numerous health benefits and a Nobel Prize.[116]

Nevertheless, it is always a plus to supply high-quality fats and proteins before and after fasting. For this reason, low-carb diets such as the keto diet have proven effective when fasting.

9. Fasting Makes You Hungry and Overeat

One widely held dietary advice is that we should never miss a meal.

The motivation for this advice is that skipping a meal could cause overeating in the following food intake.

Fortunately, studies have been conducted to give us insight into this claim with this in mind.

On the one hand, although this will indeed cause the next meal to be larger, the total energy intake remains below the result of eating all the day's regular meals.

After subjects fasted for an entire day, their caloric intake increased from 2,436 to 2,914 the next day, but in contrast, their regular overall caloric intake would have been double the first value.

That's 4,872 calories. The bottom line in food intake was a deficit of about 2,000 calories.

Beyond that, the researchers had to conclude in the context of this study that fasting could not release unconditioned cravings, as many people assume.[117]

In my experience, the body also adapts to the new rhythm of food intake during intermittent fasting, putting the size of meals into perspective.

In summary, fasting does not overwhelm you with hunger, as many people assume.

Accordingly, researchers at the University of Vienna have shown that ghrelin, the hunger hormone, steadily decreases during fasting.

When we are accustomed to ingesting food, ghrelin release increases in a pulsatile manner.

According to scientists, ghrelin causes weight gain through increased food intake and impaired fat utilization.[118]

10. Breakfast Is the Most Important

Over the years, we have learned daily routines and, with them, eating habits.

This fact is especially actual for morning hunger. Therefore, contrary to popular belief, breakfast is the most important meal of the day for the food industry but not humankind.

It is ultimately easier to reach for convenience foods when time is short.

Most people believe skipping breakfast can lead to excessive hunger, lack of concentration, and weight gain. Hence, this is one of the most persistent myths against intermittent fasting.

But otherwise, you'll lack energy for the day, right?

Not really. When we wake up in the morning, the body elevates adrenaline, glucagon, growth hormone, and cortisol levels, which provide enough energy to start the day.[119]

Therefore, it is just after waking up that it is least necessary to supply energy.

A 16-week study with 283 overweight people confirmed this by not observing weight gain in any individual skipping breakfast.[120]

However, due to the functioning of our hormone system, this result is logical. By eating breakfast, you shorten the fasting period from 16 to a maximum of 12 hours.

Therefore, insulin levels rise again earlier, leaving the body less time to burn fat for energy.

In addition, fat-burning efficiency correlates with the length of the fasting period.

Accordingly, other studies show that skipping meals can positively regulate insulin, blood glucose, abdominal fat, and body mass index.[121,122]

These are good reasons to forgo breakfast. Besides, in my experience, you'll have unlearned morning hunger in no more than two weeks anyway.

Is Intermittent Fasting Suitable for Women?

You, too, have probably read that there are unique fasting methods for women, such as crescendo fasting.

In addition, articles circulating on the Internet claim that intermittent fasting is only beneficial for men.

Nevertheless, fasting is a natural state our ancestors usually did not choose.

The fact that not only the male body is built for it is based on the fact that we exist today. For this, especially women had to survive food shortages.

However, hormonal and genetic differences between men and women play a role in intermittent fasting.

But that intermittent fasting is fundamentally unsuitable for women is a myth.

There is no question that a change in the diet affects hormonal balance. For this reason, what you eat significantly influences the phases of your menstrual cycle.

While some women report fewer symptoms of *premenstrual syndrome (PMS)* after starting intermittent fasting, others claim that fasting initially upsets their cycle.

To understand how intermittent fasting affects a woman's body, we must first understand why it can be sensitive to changes in food intake.

Sensitivity of the Female Body

Fasting affects each person differently, depending on their current state of health and other lifestyle factors, such as stress.

However, it is typical for diet and weight loss changes to affect the menstrual cycle.

Ultimately, menstruation can be sensitive to caloric restriction in particular.

When calorie intake is too low, the hypothalamus in the brain is affected.

This way, the secretion of gonadotropin-releasing hormone (GnRH) can be disrupted, which contributes to the production of two fertility hormones that we have already heard of:[123]

- Luteinizing hormone (LH)
- Follicle-stimulating hormone (FSH)

Both hormones play decisive roles in the phases of the female cycle. Therefore, drastic restrictions in food intake can affect menstruation.

Does Fasting Affect Your Period?

If the fertility hormones do not communicate appropriately with the ovaries, the period may not occur.

There are three causes of this hypothalamic interference with the period:[124]

- Excessive stress
- Excessive exercise
- Weight loss (due to excessive calorie restriction).

That intermittent fasting can upset the female cycle and is therefore not suitable for women is usually argued with the help of two rat studies since no human studies exist.

Here the rats were subjected to Alternate-Day-Fasting (ADF). And here lies the crux of the issue. Eating one day, fasting one day is for a rodent, the human equivalent of eating one week, eating nothing for one week.

Accordingly, such an extreme caloric restriction is a therapeutic fast and no longer an intermittent fast.

The first study on albino rats showed irregular cycles after excessive fasting. The long-term caloric restriction reduced the satiety hormone leptin in female rats disrupting the menstrual cycle.

As a result, kisspeptin production in the hypothalamus was inhibited. Since the peptide hormone regulates the release of GnRH, the fertility hormones LH and FSH were reduced as well.[125]

The second study showed a 31% increased chance of irregular periods in female rats subjected to the same long fasting intervals, with minimal reduction in their estrogen levels.

In contrast, periods were utterly absent in 91% of those female rats who ate daily but reduced calories by 40%. Moreover, their estrogen levels dropped markedly in the process.[126]

What we can conclude from the rodent studies is nothing new. Extreme periods of starvation and other excessive stress factors endanger the health of the offspring.

For this reason, in extreme situations, the body directs its focus away from reproduction and toward female survival.

In contrast to the rat studies, in 2017, a randomized clinical trial (much higher validity) in 100 humans did not find different health effects of ADF on women and men.

In the course of this study, in which people actually ate one day and fasted one day, the researchers investigated:[127]

- Blood pressure
- Blood sugar
- Blood lipid levels
- Insulin levels
- Insulin resistance

However, this does not mean that we can therefore lump men and women together in the context of intermittent fasting.

This chapter has gathered enough evidence to show that the female body is more sensitive to dietary changes.

This human study shows us that the intervention in the diet must be sufficiently severe to throw the female body off track.

Excessive exercise, stress, calorie reduction, and weight loss can disrupt the menstrual cycle. However, these are not particular features of intermittent fasting.

Nevertheless, many women combine intermittent fasting with severe calorie reduction and a tremendous amount of exercise when they start doing it.

Stress caused by these severe interventions and abrupt weight loss can disrupt the female cycle.

Therefore, intermittent fasting should not be confused with a conventional diet based on calorie counting.

Ultimately, the extreme calorie restrictions of diets upset the female cycle and put reproductive health at risk.[128]

In contrast, intermittent fasting is a temporal concentration of food intake to optimize your hormones for weight loss.

It does not aim to make you eat significantly less daily and starve you in the process.

For this reason, intermittent fasting methods have emerged that are better or worse suited for the more sensitive female body.

How Women Fast Safely

Nature is interested in reproduction above all other things. Therefore, the female body always focuses on the ability to produce healthy offspring that will survive and do the same.

For this reason, the female hormonal balance tends to be more sensitive to changes in diet and other external circumstances. This way, the body can adapt more quickly to external events.

For example, the hunger hormone ghrelin can rise again more quickly after a meal in women than men.

Because of these subtle yet numerous differences, intermittent fasting methods for women have been developed to provide a more gentle start.

Shorter fasting windows of 12-14 hours do not immediately upset hormonal balance and cycle. Therefore they often offer a more successful start.

Since men do not face these hurdles, they tend to have an easier time with relevant dietary changes.

Accordingly, the so-called *crescendo fasting* is the entry-level method for women.

The less extreme weekly schedule does not immediately disrupt the production of your fertility hormones and allows a smooth transition to the 16/8 method. Your starting point is a simple 12-hour fasting window.

Intermittent Fasting 12/12

Let's start with the simplest method that numerous online sources explicitly suggest for women.

It consists of fasting for 12 hours every day, of which you sleep for 8 hours. According to this, it is not so much fasting as eating within a specific time frame.

Twelve hours makes the three classic meals of the day feasible. After that, there is simply no more snacking, which is already a significant step in the right direction for most people.

For this reason, even simple 12/12 fasting can help you get emotional eating under control.

For example, stop eating after dinner at 20:00 and don't eat the next calories again until 08:00 with breakfast the following day.

Since it is easy to do, this method can be a gentle introduction to the world of intermittent fasting. In the end, you don't have to skip any meals – just give up a snacking before bed.

In 12/12 overnight fasting, the intervals are simple:

- **Fasting window:** 12 hours

- **Eating window:** 12 hours

However, this daily schedule does not take full advantage of the benefits of fasting. The longer the fasting period, the more significant the fat loss.

In addition, the health benefits of autophagy do not become apparent until about 14 hours.[129]

These facts lead us to the classic 16/8 method. It has proven to be the most sustainable guarantee of success for women because of the better balance between fasting and eating time.

Intermittent Fasting 16/8

Although various forms of intermittent fasting exist, eating within a window of 8 hours a day has proven successful, not just for women.

Classic 16/8 Intermittent Fasting is also known as the *Lean Gains Method*, *Time-Restricted Eating* or *Peak Fasting* because it allows you to gain muscle mass while losing body fat.

Therefore, this classic method of intermittent fasting is no stranger even to bodybuilders, as they have been using it for decades.

As the name time-restricted eating already reveals, this method is the mother of intermittent fasting. It gives daily a period in which may be eaten. However, strict fasting takes place during the remaining time of the day.

For example, you eat between noon and 8:00 PM, allowing the body to fast for 16 hours with an 8-hour eating period. Since you sleep 8 of the 16 fasting hours, classic intermittent fasting is more comfortable than you might think.

Depending on your daily routine and experience, modifications have also proven successful for some women. These are, for example, 14/10 or 18/6 fasting protocols.

These methods likewise represent time-restricted eating with a shorter or longer fasting window.

As you'll notice, intermittent fasting easily adapts to your particular day and body.

Nevertheless, by far the most popular intermittent fasting daily plan remains as follows:

- **Fasting window:** 16 hours
- **Eating window:** 8 hours

Before we look at why, in my experience, 16 hours of fasting per day is the ideal period for most women, I need to introduce another method.

Many consider it the best beginner method for women.

Crescendo Fasting

The crescendo method is the middle ground between the previous two fasting protocols.

In short, it is a hormone-friendly form of 16/8 intermittent fasting designed to get you started.

Instead of daily fasting, you fast on two to three non-consecutive days per week. For example, you could choose Tuesday and Thursday or Monday, Wednesday and Friday.

This way, you don't risk abruptly causing excessive caloric restriction when you start fasting.

The gradual approach allows you to test how your body and its hormonal balance react to the change.

Accordingly, you can approach your ideal fasting schedule individually in two dimensions.

On the one hand, the fasting window of the daily plan can gradually increase from 12 to 14 to 16 hours. On the other hand, the weekly plan calls for intermittent fasting only every other day when starting.

However, you can also increase this dimension slowly approaching the whole week. As a result, you get the following range of fasting intervals for crescendo fasting:

- **Fasting window:** 12-16 hours

- **Eating window:** 8-12 hours

In addition, many women also successfully limit fasting to weekdays. That way, you're not restricted on weekends, when free time and social interactions are paramount.

To avoid disrupting fertility hormone production, you should avoid intense workouts on fasting days. Instead, you can practice yoga or go for a walk if you want to get your fat-burning rolling through exercise.

Crescendo fasting gives you the advantage of doing strength training and more intense workouts on days when you're not fasting without disrupting hormone balance.

Although crescendo fasting may require a bit of planning and adjustment at first, in my experience, you'll get the hang of it quickly.

In addition, it's a great stepping stone to more advanced intermittent fasting strategies.

After no more than two weeks, you should have ramped up to three fasting days per week. Ultimately, continuity makes all the difference in successfully losing weight.

Provided you feel comfortable, you can move cautiously towards 16/8 intermittent fasting.

I think it is advisable to establish a fixed 16-hour fasting window at least on weekdays after a one-month familiarization phase.

Choose your fasting window in a way you can and will keep to it in everyday life.

If you feel first class on a full 16/8 day schedule, you can extend your fasting window to 18 hours and follow an 18/6 plan if that fits into your daily routine.

Maybe these fasting intervals sound a little complicated to you right off the bat, and you're wondering why we don't just eat one day and fast one day.

After all, you may have already read one or two success stories about it.

Can't you lose weight much faster and more efficiently? These appearances are deceptive.

Why No Alternate Day Fasting?

This method sounds extremely simple – eat one day, fast the other day:

- **Fasting window:** 24 hours (small meal).

- **Eating window:** 24 hours

However, with Alternate Day Fasting (ADF), most people eat a small meal (about 500 calories) on the fasting day.

Therefore, although it is relatively widespread, this method is not my favorite.

An incomplete meal not only makes you hungry but also negates the health benefits of autophagy. Why this cell cleansing process is so essential to the health benefits of fasting is something the following subsection will explain to us.

Besides, the 500-calorie snack also inevitably means that your body will start producing insulin again in the middle of the fasting period. And as we already know, the antilipolytic effect of insulin ensures that you won't be able to burn body fat.

If you want to lose weight and improve your health, ADF with a meal in between is not a great starting point.

So why is this fasting method so widespread?

The chances are that you have also heard from friends that they have tried ADF.

However, trying is where it stops most of the time. People try ADF, fail miserably, and give up.

It is easy to explain why the lion's share of people does not succeed in losing weight with ADF.

Most people abuse ADF because they think it allows them to maintain their unhealthy Western diet of refined carbohydrates and sugar.

Many even think they have to reward themselves with junk food on eating days.

I hope I don't have to explain further that this shot can only backfire.

Moreover, poor food choices can more easily cause unpleasant side effects in the gastrointestinal tract, making it harder to stick to fasting.

For these reasons, ADF is more difficult for most people to incorporate into their daily routines than other methods.

If we remember again that the female body can be sensitive to extreme restrictions, with irregularity to boot, ADF is the wrong method for women.

You can lose weight with ADF without a snack if you don't overdo it on meal days. However, with up to 36 hours of strict caloric restriction, you run the risk of upsetting your cycle.[130]

If PMS also exacerbates cravings on a fasting day, you will wish you had chosen a less radical method.

For these reasons, time-restricted eating works better for women. 16/8 has a continuity that you can trust. You get to eat every day and never get over-whelmed by hunger.

I would also not recommend ADF to men because they will not follow the extreme fasting window either.

This fasting plan is hardly feasible in the long run and, therefore, especially unsuitable for beginners.

Should You Avoid the 5:2 Diet?

In the 5:2 diet, the calorie intake is limited to 500 calories per day for two days per week (with two meals of 250 calories each).

The fasting interval of the classic 5:2 diet is composed as follows:

- **Fasting window:** 2×1 day (small meal).

- **Eating window:** 5 days of the week

You eat regularly the remaining five days of the week. For example, you could eat only 500 calories daily on Tuesday and Friday and eat as usual on Monday, Wednesday, Thursday, Saturday, and Sunday.

For this reason, on the 5:2 diet, you practice a 36-hour fast twice a week with a small meal in the middle of the fasting window.

Although small meals may seem easier to approach fasting at first, they ruin your results.

As the meal elevates insulin levels, fat burning, autophagy, and the associated positive effects are interrupted.

In addition, a small meal cannot satiate you and will ignite hunger. The recipe for cravings afterward is perfect if it is a meal that raises blood sugar, such as bread or cereal.

Since the hunger hormone ghrelin decreases with a longer fasting duration, it is wiser to fast without the snack.[131]

Therefore, it is better to fast through the two days and boost ketosis strictly. In addition, it is even more efficient for cell renewal to fast for two days at a stretch.

But therein lies the crux of the method.

This vast calorie restriction may affect your menstrual cycle if you don't eat for 60 hours straight once a week.

Fasting periods of more than 36 hours can put additional stress on the female body. In such situations, it may declare survival its primary goal instead of fertility.

No other intermittent fasting method can so quickly induce hypothalamic amenorrhea, the absence of menstruation.

If you exercise as well, the likelihood is even higher.[132]

If, on the other hand, you practice 5:2 fasting with snacks in between, the success is moderate, and the cravings are enormous.

In my experience, 16/8 fasting is much more efficient for women. You don't have to starve yourself, your cycle doesn't go off track immediately, and you lose weight continuously and sustainably.

No drastic restrictions, stress, and abrupt weight loss help keep your hormones balanced.

Why 16 Hours of Fasting Work

Now that we have analyzed various intermittent fasting methods, you may wonder why a fasting period of 16 hours would work best.

Wouldn't the effect of intermittent fasting inevitably increase in effectiveness with the duration of the fasting window?

With this in mind, wouldn't methods with more extended fasting periods such as *One Meal a Day (OMAD)* be more appropriate?

The reason for 16/8's success story is the balance of several key factors that are critical to successful fasting:

- Practical benefits in everyday life
- Effective fat burning
- Activation of autophagy

On the one hand, there are practical reasons for the 16 hours of intermittent fasting. If you skip breakfast or dinner, you extend the natural fasting window. This way, you reach the 16 hours of intermittent fasting without much effort.

For a good reason, you might have heard that people lose weight while sleeping because that is the last fasting time we have left, thanks to conventional dietary advice.[133]

Eating from 12:00 p.m. to 8:00 p.m. is enormously comfortable because morning hunger is learned. You will realize this fact no later than two weeks after starting the 16/8 method.

During this time, most people unlearn their morning hunger.

Besides, our body injects us with a cocktail of hormones in the morning, which provides enough energy for the day ahead, as we know by now.

Moreover, skipping breakfast allows us to always have dinner with the family. Since dinner is an essential social cornerstone of many families, this variant can be comfortably integrated into everyday life than others.

Nevertheless, it doesn't mean you have to skip breakfast. You can also do 16/8 intermittent fasting by skipping dinner. Finally, intermittent fasting is flexible, and you can adapt it to your daily routine.

Unlike these two variants, skipping lunch is less effective.

Why is that?

This question brings us to two other factors that make a powerful argument for 16 hours of daily fasting.

Fat burning and autophagy require low insulin since it's also one of the three essential nutrient sensors in the human body.

Although weight loss also causes health benefits, most of the positive effects of fasting in our bodies are supported by autophagy.

Because this recycling process in human cells is responsible for breakthrough health benefits of fasting, its discovery was even honored with the Nobel Prize in Medicine.[134]

According to recent studies, humans need at least 14 hours without meals to activate autophagy in their bodies significantly.[135]

However, a low baseline level of autophagy exists at all times because it is our body's maintenance service.

Therefore, it is not immediately activated or deactivated 100% as with a switch.

Even though the process is very individual and difficult to measure, two hours of cell cleansing is remarkable if we consider that the anti-aging effect is repeated daily and eventually adds up.

However, you can speed up the process by exercising and eating a low-carbohydrate diet, increasing autophagy's effectiveness during the 16 hours.

Thus, we have found the third essential argument for 16 hours of intermittent fasting.

Accordingly, 16/8 intermittent fasting is the perfect trade-off for maximizing weight loss, convenience, and health benefits that have been proven over years of experimentation.

Now let's look in detail at why, in my experience, the method works best for most women.

Practical Benefits

Although many women come across 16/8 intermittent fasting because they want to lose weight in the short term, they often stick with it in the long run because of the practical benefits.

Unlike most other methods, 16/8 is a lifestyle you can effortlessly establish for the long term.

In addition, it provides more energy, better concentration, and therefore more productivity at work.

Thus, after a few weeks or even days, most beginners find that intermittent fasting makes their lives easier.

In contrast to the health benefits to which we will turn, few people say a word about the practical benefits of this diet.

The following benefits in everyday life significantly distinguish intermittent fasting from conventional diets.

While most diets overwhelm you with countless workouts, complicated recipes, tedious portioning, calorie counting, and tracking, 16/8 helps you minimize your daily effort.

1. Fasting Is Incredibly Simple

Unlike most dietary advice, intermittent fasting is simple for beginners. Classic 16/8 intermittent fasting has two rules:

- No breakfast
- No snacks

The bottom line, the simpler the rules, the easier it is to implement methods in everyday life.

2. It's Surprisingly Cheap

Intermittent fasting is not only free, but it also saves you money. Accordingly, you won't need the following things to have success with fasting:

- Breakfast
- Processed food
- Expensive exotic superfoods
- A gym subscription

Even though fitness, pharmaceutical, and food marketing have taught us contradictorily, less is usually better. You'll realize this effect in your checking account.

3. Intermittent Fasting Saves Lots of Time

The food industry loves diet advice that involves multiple meals since no one can cook six times a day. This way, they create more demand for convenience foods.

On the other hand, intermittent fasting allows you to focus on one or two meals and prepare them relaxed using real food or skip a meal if there is no time.

This way, you save yourself the junk food, the food coma after eating, and time and money on stressful days.

4. Fasting Is Possible With Any Diet

Intermittent fasting 16/8 is not a trendy special diet but a refrain.

Since fasting is about the time when you don't eat anything, you don't need new recipe collections and shopping lists.

That's why you can start intermittent fasting today if you:

- Are a vegetarian
- Eat animal products
- Do not eat wheat
- Are lactose intolerant
- Are shopping on a budget
- Are on the go all-day

- Allergic to nuts

- Are 80 years old

- Do not like cooking

- Are a top chef

In short, hardly anything can stop you from starting intermittent fasting today.

5. You Can Do It Always and Everywhere

Beginners do not need special knowledge or preparation for intermittent fasting.

Besides, you don't have to buy anything to start fasting finally. You can do it anytime and anywhere by simply skipping a meal.

As an intermittent fasting beginner, you only need resolution, water, tea, or coffee.

6. Intermittent Fasting Can Reduce Stress

Unlike diets, fasting does not involve more effort but always less.

And that also affects the levels of your primary stress hormone, cortisol. When the diet adds to an already stressful daily routine, it doesn't help you relax.

For example, you can use the time you gain to read a book or exercise. Conventional diets probably can't offer this advantage.

Effective Fat Burning

There is a good reason why people can achieve outstanding weight loss results with intermittent fasting. Fasting is the most effective way to lower insulin levels.

Insulin blocks the enzyme that breaks down body fat and, in turn, promotes the activity of the enzyme that builds body fat.[136,137]

Accordingly, researchers can now predict about 75% of possible gains and losses in overweight people using insulin levels.[138]

Moreover, diabetes studies can tell us that insulin is the essential regulator of body weight.

Type 2 diabetes is usually treated with intensified insulin therapy.

And what is the side effect par excellence? Weight gain!

A randomized controlled trial at the Oxford Center for Diabetes, Endocrinology, and Metabolism compared insulin treatments.

Subjects on low doses gained an average of 1.9 kilograms, those on medium gained 4.7 kilograms, and those on high doses gained 5.7 kilograms.[139]

Similarly, numerous other studies provide the same evidence: the general side effect of insulin is weight gain.[140]

Intermittent fasting can help restore the natural balance between eating and fasting, thereby normalizing insulin levels.

A 16-hour fasting window cuts off the nutrient intake, lowers insulin levels, and thus ends the fat storage mode in the body.

The body can then begin to break down carbohydrates stored in the form of glycogen. Once glycogen stores are empty, body fat can be burned for energy.[141]

This process of efficient fat burning is called ketosis and, contrary to many myths, is an entirely natural mechanism that has ensured the survival of our species.

During ketosis, the liver converts fatty acids into ketones or ketone bodies, which your body can use more efficiently as a source of energy.

Nature designed the body to build up fat reserves in times of abundance to draw on this body fat in food shortages.

For this reason, the term winter fat evolved, as body fat was burned for energy in the winter when food was unavailable.

Therefore, a keto diet also attempts to put the body into ketosis by depriving it of carbohydrates, which in nature could initially only be achieved by fasting.[142]

Because today, instead of food shortages, we experience an endless summer and eat around the clock daily, we gain weight.

The 16/8 method gives your body two-thirds of the day to set the hormonal course back to effective weight loss.

Because you sleep half of it and still get to eat half of the day (eight hours), this fasting window became easy to obey.

No other method fits into a daily routine so quickly while still providing maximum comfort.

Autophagy Activation

The third primary driver of intermittent fasting's popularity is its myriad health benefits.

In addition to weight loss, autophagy is predominantly responsible for the rejuvenating effects of fasting.

Autophagy is a mechanism in our bodies that sorts out or recycles discarded organelles, proteins, and cell membranes.

Autophagy kicks in when there is no longer enough energy to sustain decayed cellular parts.

It's an orderly process of degradation and recycling of cellular components.

For this reason, autophagy means self-eating if we translate it.

In this context, autophagy has three essential tasks in our cells:

- Remove defective proteins and organelles
- Eliminate pathogens
- Prevent atypical protein accumulation

When food is scarce, the body goes from growth mode to maintenance mode. It then launches this intracellular recycling system that breaks down broken cell parts and directs toxins out of the body.

In this way, autophagy prevents modern diseases that plague us today. For example, these are cancer, diabetes, cardiovascular disease, polycystic ovary syndrome, Parkinson's disease, and Alzheimer's disease.[143,144,145,146,147]

For this reason, the term autophagy was accompanied by two Nobel Prize winners at once.

After discovering that lysosomes can break down cell components, the Belgian biochemist Christian de Duve was the first to coin the term autophagy.

He was also awarded the Nobel Prize in 1974 for this fundamental finding.

But a Japanese scientist started the decisive experiments in the early 1990s on yeast cells.

Consequently, Yoshinori Ohsumi's work showed precisely how the processes involved in autophagy work and how crucial they are for health.

Therefore, he was awarded the Nobel Prize in Medicine in 2016 for discovering this mechanism activated by fasting.

Accordingly, Yoshinori Ohsumi named his Nobel lecture: *Autophagy – an Intracellular Recycling System.*[148]

But how is autophagy activated?

For this purpose, three essential nutrient sensors exist in our bodies. Simply put, they turn the process of autophagy on and off:

- **Insulin:** Sensitive to carbohydrates and proteins.

- **mTOR:** Sensitive to proteins

- **AMPK:** Sensitive to lack of energy in cells

AMP-activated protein kinase (AMPK) responds when cells are supplied with energy, regardless of the macronutrient delivered. Therefore, in addition to carbohydrates and proteins, fat also inhibits autophagy.

AMPK and insulin also activate *mTOR, the mechanistic or mammalian target of rapamycin.*

Therefore, this enzyme, which is essential for growth, is called the primary nutrient sensor in our body. As soon as you eat, it detects nutrient availability and inhibits autophagy.

Therefore, even a tiny amount of glucose or amino acids can interfere with autophagy.

For this reason, autophagy only occurs during genuine fasting. Simple caloric restriction or dieting cannot activate autophagy.

By causing the nutrient sensors to kick in, we signal our body to grow.

Therefore, nutrient sensors stop autophagy because it is a *catabolic (breaking down)*, not an *anabolic (building up)* mechanism.

Accordingly, excess nutrients put the body into growth mode via mTOR. On the other hand, fasting – the absence of nutrients – puts our body into natural maintenance mode.

In this process, the body acts sustainably and pulls defective cell parts to produce energy or build new organelles.

Now that we've discussed the processes that initiate them, it's time to learn about the intermittent fasting benefits critical for health.

Health Benefits for Women

Fasting sets in motion impressive processes in our bodies. Thanks to recent advances in biochemistry and medicine, we increasingly gain groundbreaking insights into the effects of fasting.

Here are the most critical health benefits of intermittent fasting for women that research can explain to date:

1. Anti-Aging Effect

Every vehicle must be cared for and regularly maintained to function in excellent quality for as long as possible.

Therefore, fasting is the best way to keep your body in shape through autophagy.[149]

Once this intracellular recycling system is at work, it prevents the diseases that plague our Western society:

- Dementia, Alzheimer's and Parkinson's[150]
- Muscle and bone atrophy[151]
- Cardiovascular diseases[152]
- Insulin resistance and type 2 diabetes[153]
- Cancer[154]

In addition, research is increasingly unraveling

that autophagy is also likely to renew damaged proteins and organelles in cardiac cells.[155]

Moreover, since it can generally slow down the aging process, autophagy is probably the most convincing reason to fast for at least 14 hours.[156]

2. Reduced Inflammation

Aging is the accumulation of cellular damage with a decreasing ability to repair it. As a result, aging fundamentally causes some degree of inflammation in the body.

Recent studies suggest fasting-induced autophagy can significantly slow this aging process and increase lifespan.[157]

Therefore, intermittent fasting also achieves remarkable results in treating age-related diseases.

Moreover, intermittent fasting can reduce the need for proteins in the diet, as the body recycles proteins from broken cell parts. This fact again has a positive effect on longevity.

Against this background, widespread modern diseases such as arteriosclerosis, cancer, or type 2 diabetes are characterized by too much growth and proteins.

In addition to autophagy, which breaks down defective proteins and protein accumulation, reducing inflammation in the body contributes to increased longevity.

Furthermore, ketosis during fasting lowers blood sugar and insulin levels, reducing inflammation and free radicals in the body that cause disease.

Therefore, another recent study notes that intermittent fasting directly causes an increase in life expectancy.[158]

3. Increased Energy

Mitochondria are our cells' tiny power plants. They metabolize energy from food into the universally usable energy carrier *adenosine triphosphate (ATP)*.

Accordingly, it is hardly surprising that many mitochondria exist in metabolic organs such as the liver.

Fasting induces mitophagy, autophagy at the level of mitochondria.

As a result, the body breaks down older and non-functioning mitochondria to produce new and healthy mitochondria. This process improves cellular energy availability and metabolic flexibility.

Furthermore, this quality control of mitochondria protects against stress, heart disease, and the progression of malignant tumor cells.[159]

Moreover, this counteracting of aging processes promotes cellular rejuvenation.

In addition, human studies can demonstrate measurable increases in energy levels from even short periods of fasting.

Using a smartphone app, researchers have determined that the average person's natural fasting window coincides with time spent in bed.

That means most people eat throughout their entire waking hours.

When the researchers shortened the eating window of overweight subjects to 10 to 11 hours a day, they noted more energy, improved sleep, and weight loss.[160]

4. Improved Cognition

In the brain, too, intermittent fasting can help break down accumulations of toxic proteins that promote dementia.

Accordingly, scientists found that in the early stages of dementia, the process of autophagy is significantly low.[161]

However, if ketones are burned from the fat stores instead of glucose from the carbohydrate stores through fasting or working out, signaling pathways increasing learning and memory function are activated.

Intermittent fasting can thus counteract neurodegenerative diseases such as Parkinson's or Alzheimer's.[162]

One of these signal generators is the neuronal growth hormone BDNF (brain-derived neurotrophic factor), responsible for forming new nerve cells.

Therefore, high BDNF levels are also associated with increased intelligence and memory function.

When you release BDNF, your brain can form new neural connections. For example, according to studies, fasting could improve memory in older people.[163]

In this context, the sympathetic nervous system is also activated, and the body releases adrenaline, cortisol, and growth hormones.

For this reason, many people report increased cognition and alertness when fasting.

Hence, studies have not found a reduction in cognition in people who fasted for two days straight.[164]

Only breaking the fast allows the body to relax. Thus, the mental focus also fades again. You may have already noticed this circumstance as sluggishness after the meal.

5. Antidepressant Effect

Countless clinical observations point to an antidepressant effect of fasting, sometimes even accompanied by euphoria.

According to a recent meta-analysis, patients

consistently reported improvement in three essential factors:[165]

- Mood
- Alertness
- Serenity

According to the researchers, who generally classify fasting as safe, various neurobiological mechanisms could be responsible for this.

These include changes in neurotransmitters, sleep quality, and the synthesis of neurotrophic factors, such as BDNF.

6. Boosted Metabolism

Contrary to the myth that intermittent fasting slows down metabolism, scientists have long proven that it boosts it instead.[166]

Because fasting releases growth hormones and adrenaline, our ancestors could forage longer for food, precisely when it was scarce.

That's why they were able to ensure the species' survival even during food shortages.[167]

Consequently, intermittent fasting increases your body's efficiency in tapping into stored fat for energy.

In addition, the release of hormones such as norepinephrine keeps the basal metabolic rate up.[168]

7. Improved Muscle Gain

Intermittent fasting is no stranger to bodybuilding either. Classic time-restricted eating, in which you do not eat for 14 to 18 hours daily, is a proven method to gain lean mass.

Thereby, it is crucial to work out in a fasted state. Exercising on an empty stomach promotes not only autophagy but also fat burning.

Contrary to popular belief, muscles do not atrophy at all during fasting.

As we have already heard, intermittent fasting increases the release of growth hormones.

Thus, during fasting, not only muscle but also bone mass is protected from degeneration.[169]

Accordingly, targeted intermittent fasting combined with appropriate training is an effective natural method for improved muscle gains.[170]

8. Enhanced Fat Burning

Intermittent fasting aims to burn fat as a primary energy source during the fasting periods.

When released fatty acids from body fat or food enter the liver, they are converted into ketones to provide energy for the body. This metabolic process is therefore called ketosis.

Hence, fasting is the ultimate ketogenic diet because the body can only obtain energy from body fat without food intake.

For this reason, ketosis induced by intermittent fasting can burn fat reserves remarkably quickly.[171]

Furthermore, ketosis helps regulate appetite and stabilize blood sugar, supporting intermittent fasting and weight loss.

Accordingly, ketone energy does not cause blood sugar to spike as it does after high-carbohydrate meals. In addition, because ketones can cross the blood-brain barrier, they can provide sustained, clean mental energy.[172]

9. Less Visceral Fat

Intermittent fasting not only burns visually unflattering fat deposits.

Against this background, current studies state that intermittent fasting burns dangerous visceral fat more effectively than low-carb diets.[173]

Visceral fat deposits are fat accumulations in and around vital organs, such as the liver, intestines, or pancreas. There they lay the origin of secondary diseases.

Intra-organic fat contributes to non-alcoholic fatty liver disease, type 2 diabetes, and cardiovascular disease.[174]

Since the liver is the first place where malignant fat accumulates, it is often the root of modern metabolic diseases such as insulin resistance.

10. Improved Insulin Sensitivity

The scientific record of the effect of fasting on insulin resistance dates back to 1969.[175]

Also, today, studies refer to intermittent fasting as a safe treatment for insulin resistance.[176]

Insulin resistance is a protective mechanism against the vast amounts of insulin caused by the *Wester Pattern Diet (WPD)*, dominated by refined carbohydrates.

In this process, cells no longer respond appropriately to insulin, which prevents them from absorbing sufficient glucose from the bloodstream.

However, fat cells cannot become insulin resistant and blithely store energy. Therefore, obesity is a significant symptom of the disease.

Besides combating the causative hyperinsulinemia, intermittent fasting can also reduce insulin resistance in the cells.

Thus, fasting can reverse type 2 diabetes, the most significant secondary disease of insulin resistance, which diets alone usually cannot do.[177]

11. Increased Fertility

While excessive fasting may pose a threat for some women, properly executed intermittent fasting can positively affect fertility.

Polycystic ovarian syndrome (PCOS) is women's most common metabolic disorder. It characterizes the development of cysts on the ovaries based on hormonal imbalance.

Like type 2 diabetes, polycystic ovary syndrome is often characterized by obesity, hypertension, and insulin resistance.[178]

Nevertheless, in a recent study, intermittent fasting was able to help overweight women with PCOS. Because fasting increases the release of luteinizing hormone, it helps promote ovulation.

Furthermore, fasting, weight loss, and improved mental health may contribute to fertility.[179]

12. Enhanced Tissue Regeneration

Intermittent fasting works against age-related loss of tissue function.

That's according to a recent study by researchers at Harvard University and the Massachusetts Institute of Technology (MIT).

They showed that short-term fasting helps improve stem cell function by initiating a fat-burning process.

Therefore, they conclude that intermittent fasting is a viable strategy to improve tissue regeneration, particularly intestinal tissue.[180]

13. Improved Gut Health

Intermittent fasting is one of the best ways to improve gut health.

On the one hand, fasting periods allow the intestines to rest; on the other hand, they starve out harmful gut bacteria.

But already, shorter fasting periods work. A current study suggests that an improved life expectancy due to short intermittent fasting periods at a young age is determined.

In particular, reducing inflammation, which often has its origin in the gut, slows down the aging process.

Accordingly, intermittent fasting also reduces age-related diseases and strengthens the intestinal wall.[181]

Other studies go even further, suggesting that intermittent fasting helps repair intestinal permeability, also known as *leaky gut*.[182]

Furthermore, intermittent fasting has the positive side effect of improving food intolerances.

14. Boosted Immune System

Defects in the immune system are significant drivers of aging and disease development.

Researchers showed that fasting could alter stem cells to promote stress resistance, self-renewal, and regeneration.[183]

Intermittent fasting also improves metabolic profiles and reduces the risk of obesity and resulting diseases such as nonalcoholic fatty liver disease and chronic diseases such as diabetes and cancer.[184]

Fewer meals per day can counteract disease processes and improve a variety of age-related as well as Alzheimer's, Parkinson's, and cardiovascular diseases.[185]

15. Improved Sleep-Wake Rhythm

Humans have evolved an internal clock that ensures that physiological processes in the body occur at the right times.[186]

These so-called *circadian rhythms* occur in a 24-hour sleep-wake cycle and influence behavior and physical health, such as the gut flora.[187]

Food intake is the most crucial zeitgeber for circadian rhythm function. Therefore, it controls physiological, behavioral, and metabolic processes.[188]

When these circadian rhythms are disrupted, for example, by constant snacking, metabolism is negatively affected.

Obesity, type 2 diabetes, cardiovascular disease, and cancer are the long-term consequences of jet lag induced by eating behaviors.[189,190]

Intermittent fasting can help synchronize circadian rhythms, leading to reprogramming metabolism and subsequently natural regulation of hormone balance and body weight.

An intact sleep-wake rhythm is vital for optimizing health and life expectancy.

How Intermittent Fasting Helps with PMS

The hormonal transition from ovulation to the proliferation phase of the next cycle can affect mood, cognitive and physical health.[191]

According to studies, premenstrual syndrome (PMS) affects 47.8% of women of reproductive age worldwide.[192]

At least 80-90% of women experience some sign of PMS at some point.[193]

Doesn't intermittent fasting then affect physical and mental health all the more?

Yes, but intermittent fasting can alleviate PMS symptoms rather than exacerbate them.

The prerequisite is balanced fasting plans, such as 16/8, and physical activity that remains within a healthy range, not putting additional stress on the female body.

Here are five ways that appropriate intermittent fasting can help you with PMS symptoms.

1. Mood and Cravings

One of the most common PMS symptoms is cravings. Whether it's sweets, salty snacks, or fat, many women feel out of control when eating during their period.

Targeted intermittents of fasting can help with cravings in several ways.

For example, in a study of uncontrolled eating behaviors, intermittent fasting significantly reduced cravings and depression after only two months. In addition, fasting positively affected participants' body image perception.[194]

The balance between eating and fasting also stabilizes blood sugar levels, often responsible for cravings for sweets, as a new study in which subjects underwent 18/6-intermittent fasting confirms.

In addition to improved blood sugar regulation, the researchers noted anti-aging effects and increased BDNF levels.[195]

Brain-derived neurotrophic factor (BDNF) is a neuronal growth hormone that forms new neural connections in the brain.[196]

Therefore, it stands to reason that intermittent fasting for PMS symptoms could improve mood and cognition in general.

2. Estrogen

Improved blood glucose levels also result in better insulin levels. Finally, glucose is the primary stimulus of insulin secretion.

Insulin is the critical hormone for weight loss and essential for sex hormone balance. Thus, no stone is left unturned when hormone balance gets out of whack.

Excessively high insulin levels make people fat and inhibit the production of *sex hormone-binding globulin (SHBG)* in the liver.[197]

SHBG's role is to bind estrogen in the blood, keeping it balanced. As a result, excessively high insulin levels impair estrogen levels and thus also the female cycle.

Also, a healthy estrogen level is essential for cognitive thinking.[198]

Furthermore, a study of more than 100 overweight women showed that intermittent fasting for six months could lower insulin levels by nearly one-third and increase insulin sensitivity.[199]

According to this fact, intermittent fasting can further support your hormone balance and help prevent type 2 diabetes.

3. Sleep

Intermittent fasting can help with PMS symptoms such as lack of sleep

Women whose hormones are out of balance experience difficulties falling asleep or sleeping through the night.

If you've ever struggled with sleep issues, you know that one night of poor sleep can ruin your entire next day.

Accordingly, recent studies state that the impact of sleep quality on mood is dramatically higher than the other way round.[200]

On the other hand, intermittent fasting can help significantly improve sleep quality, according to a study conducted on 14 women and one man.

After just one week of intermittent fasting, the participants were already able to observe the following improvements in their sleep patterns:[201]

- Reduced awakenings
- Fewer leg movements
- Longer REM sleep
- Improved sleep quality
- Increased energy level
- Improved concentration
- Emotional balance

Hence, a regulated eating window, e.g., between noon and 8:00 p.m., is now considered an attractive strategy for synchronizing sleep-wake rhythms to improve sleep hygiene.[202]

4. Concentration

Nothing is more frustrating than sitting down to work and having a hard time concentrating. Hormone imbalance, particularly estrogen dominance, can lead to cognitive impairments such as brain fog.

As we just heard, the positive effects of intermittent fasting on sleep quality can improve daytime concentration.[203]

But that's not all. Fasting can increase neural network activity in cognitive brain regions, leading to BDNF production, improved neural adaptation, and stress tolerance.[204]

Accordingly, some people report improved memory, concentration, and learning ability during intermittent fasting.

This hypothesis is corroborated by a study in which subjects ate only between 08:00 and 14:00, significantly increasing their BDNF release.[205]

5. Inflammation

Researchers in California have found that the following PMS symptoms are significantly related to increased levels of inflammation in the body:[206]

- Mood swings
- Abdominal cramps
- Back pain
- Loss of appetite
- Weight gain
- Bloating
- Chest pain

At least since the discovery of autophagy, fasting has been known to counteract inflammation in the body and diseases based on it.[207]

Accordingly, numerous studies show intermittent fasting can lower inflammatory markers contributing to weight gain and insulin resistance.[208]

Thus, intermittent fasting can help to alleviate inflammation-induced PMS symptoms naturally.

Potential Side Effects

Most people are used to burning only sugar for energy because of the Western Pattern Diet (WPD). Therefore, switching to fat burning for the first time can bring the following symptoms:

- Headache
- Dizziness
- Low motivation
- Nausea
- Stomach pain

These physical symptoms are also known as the *keto flu* because the ketogenic diet requires the body to get used to burning fat for energy in the same way.

The trigger for this is the depletion of carbohydrate stores. Before the body can go into ketosis, it preferentially consumes glucose from glycogen in the liver and skeletal muscles.

Glycogen is a branched multisugar, with about two to three grams of water for every gram of carbohydrate.

Since this causes the body to flush out a lot of water and electrolytes, physical symptoms, notably headaches, and dizziness, can occur.

However, these disappear permanently once the body is fat-adapted. Hence, the body has gained metabolic flexibility and can burn fat for primary energy in addition to glucose.

In addition, keto flu can be prevented during intermittent fasting if you have the right practical hints, which I will share in the book's third central part.

Is Fasting Safe for Any Woman?

Although many beginners achieve immediate success with intermittent fasting, it is not necessarily suitable for all individuals.

Accordingly, there are situations when intermittent fasting may be inappropriate. Therefore, fasting can be a problem in the following conditions:

- **Chronic stress:** Although healthy can be stressful, there are times in life when Intermittent Fasting can be the straw that breaks the camel's back. If you're currently going through a mentally challenging phase of your life, focus on stress relief instead.

- **Eating disorders:** Self-care is also needed when you try Intermittent Fasting. Return to a standardized eating plan when you develop a questionable relationship with food. Fasting may not suit you if you have a history of anorexia or another eating disorder.

In addition to these situations, many women ask themselves the exciting question of whether they can practice intermittent fasting during pregnancy.

Can a time-restricted eating window be dangerous when the female body undergoes numerous changes?

Intermittent Fasting and Pregnancy

After many women ask themselves whether it is safe to practice intermittent fasting during pregnancy, there is a general answer.

Always talk to your doctor before making any significant changes to your diet.

If we consider that intermittent fasting promotes weight loss and limits growth, a controversy about pregnancy arises.

Pregnancy, on the other hand, has different goals than fasting:

- **Weight gain** of the child
- **Growth** in a short time

Since the goals could hardly be more opposite, it surprises little that nobody will straight recommend intermittent fasting while a woman is pregnant.

Beyond that, too few studies could give well-founded recommendations on whether intermittent fasting has positive or negative effects on the pregnancy.

Furthermore, no studies are targeting intermittent fasting during the entire pregnancy.

Aggravating is that studies about fasting while pregnancy are limited to Ramadan.

During this religious type of intermittent fasting, one does not eat from sunrise to sunset. In contrast to intermittent fasting for health benefits, you eat right before and after sleep.

With this in mind, the significance of these studies for intermittent fasting decreases.

However, these studies on Ramadan fasting while pregnancy suggest that the following characteristics are not influenced by the fast:[209,210]

- Birth Weight
- Premature births

Although these investigations do not suggest any adverse effects of fasting on pregnancy, the researchers agree that there is still far too little data to conclude.

Moreover, we must note that the Islamic fasting custom excludes pregnant women. Nevertheless, many of them do fast voluntarily.

However, it is interesting that a current study could determine the reduced risk of gestational diabetes and obesity by fasting in the second trimester.[211]

Is Fasting Safe During Pregnancy?

Although we struggle with these diseases of too much growth and proteins, there are still phases in life where growth is the main focus. And pregnancy is an essential one of them.

Accordingly, two lives require more energy and protein than just one.

Increased ketone levels of pregnant women support this fact. The body mobilizes energy from fat reserves if insufficient power is available to ensure a child's healthy growth.[212]

Therefore, pregnancy is a period that has unique priorities:

- Nutrient supply for healthy body development
- Exceptional growth and weight gain in a short time
- Evolution of maternal fat reserves for breastfeeding

Likewise, the purpose of breast milk in all mammals stresses out these growth and weight gain goals.

Against this background, dramatically changing eating habits can lead to nutrient deficiencies.

Moreover, fasting can change the hormone balance. For example, the release of norepinephrine is increased, which is not ideal during rest.[213]

On top of that, human bodies are individual. Thus fasting can have different effects. Therefore nothing can replace the personal exchange with a doctor you trust.

Therefore apparent alternatives arise in pregnancy:

- Working out an individual plan for healthy weight gain with the help of medical professionals

- Listening to your body, as it is always striving for the nutrients it needs (except the addictive effect of sugar)

Risks of Fasting During Pregnancy

During pregnancy, you already have enough on your mind. Therefore a strict fasting protocol would probably only increase the stress.

If you do not take care of yourself, you risk not providing your child with the high-quality food it needs.

Above all, long-term effects are largely unclear due to a lack of appropriate research.

While some Ramadan fasting studies claim to affect fetal respiration, others say there is no link between fasting and child health.[214,215]

With this in mind, we must conclude that rigorous intermittent fasting during pregnancy should be treated as a risk.

Ultimately, adequate nutrient supply for mother and child has priority.

For example, iron deficiency is a problem in pregnant women, as the iron requirement increases exponentially due to the fetus. Accordingly, potential anemia threatens both the child and the mother.[216]

Adequate intake of minerals from natural food can minimize such risks. In iron deficiency, eating liver can prevent iron deficiency.

How Fasting Can Help You Get Pregnant

Furthermore, in our context, it is interesting to note that restoring the balance between eating and fasting has been shown to affect fertility positively.

Accordingly, in overweight women with *polycystic ovary syndrome (PCOS)*, intermittent fasting was found to increase luteinizing hormone, which helps promote ovulation.

In this context, fasting's weight loss and mental health could contribute to fertility.[217]

PCOS often goes hand-in-hand with obesity, insulin resistance, or even type 2 diabetes.[218]

Some studies even suggest that insulin resistance plays the central role in the development of

PCOS, which also dramatically increases the risk of diabetes in young women.[219]

Intermittent Fasting Before Pregnancy

Since it can increase fertility, intermittent fasting seems reasonably practicable, as far as still no pregnancy is suspected.

If you do intermittent fasting before pregnancy to increase a future mother's health, you might reap significant benefits while pregnant.

When we look at the critical health benefits of intermittent fasting, that can make sense:

- Increased insulin sensitivity
- Reduced inflammation
- Improved metabolism
- Increased fat burning
- Improved gut health

However, when getting pregnant, even experienced fasting enthusiasts should individually discuss the topic with a professional. She might even allow you to continue mild fasting due to your condition.

Alternatives to Intermittent Fasting

That you cannot continue fasting precisely the same way does not mean that you have to neglect your diet during pregnancy.

That's why you can always focus on healthy fats and avoid refined carbohydrates during your meals.

For example, this means reducing sweets, bread, and other bakery and instead including grass-fed butter, virgin coconut oil, or avocados into your diet.

Simultaneously, this mild keto-style fat fasting can keep you fuller for longer and prevent gestational diabetes without having to forego adequate nutrient intake.

Nevertheless, you need not be ashamed of eating more during pregnancy. Excessing 200-400 calories daily is relatively standard in a healthy pregnancy.

However, even during pregnancy, you should prefer natural foods and gratefully reject processed foods with colorful packaging.

You may feel lethargic and dirty, especially in the first few months. Although this may sound controversial, exercise can improve the condition.

Furthermore, adequate physical exercise improves insulin sensitivity and reduces the risk of gestational diabetes.[220]

Exercise can even reduce the risk of cesarean section delivery.[221]

If you have been exercising regularly before pregnancy, this is ideal. Nevertheless, even in this case, you must ask your doctor if you need to change your exercise routine.

If you want to get some exercise in your life right now, walking, cycling, or swimming in moderate units (up to 45 minutes) might be suitable, provided your doctor approves this.

Nevertheless, the female body is not a machine. Whether you feel physically or mentally overwhelmed before, after, or during pregnancy, don't be afraid to seek professional help.

The bottom line is that pregnancy is not an ideal time to experiment. If you haven't tried intermittent fasting before, you shouldn't start, especially during pregnancy.

However, it doesn't last forever either.

If you want to try intermittent fasting, post-delivery is a better time. If your doctor gives you the go, you can lose weight more efficiently and improve your health.

Intermittent Fasting Post Pregnancy

That you should not overdo intermittent fasting during pregnancy does not mean that you cannot find back into your fasting plan afterward.

However, after the strains of birth, there is no

question that you cannot immediately go from 0 to 100 again. And if you are breastfeeding, you must discuss this intention with your doctor.

Nevertheless, intermittent fasting post-pregnancy can help you to regain first-class health.

As studies have shown, intermittent fasting helps:[222]

- Burn fat more effectively
- Lose weight more easily
- Improve blood lipids
- Fight hypertension

Furthermore, women who practiced intermittent fasting could witness mental benefits.

Female subjects in a recent study experienced a noticeably more robust sense of achievement, pride, and control.[223]

PART III: LIFESTYLE

Clean vs. Dirty Fasting

Opinion on intermittent fasting is often not unanimous.

While some experts recommend drinking only water during the fast, others claim that low-calorie drinks, sweeteners, cream, or even Bulletproof Coffee are fine.

Clean and dirty fasting refers to whether a drink or food can technically break the fast during the fasting period.

To help us understand the difference between clean and dirty intermittent fasting based on science, we must delve deeper into the terminology.

Clean Intermittent Fasting

You don't consume any caloric foods or beverages during the 16 hours of clean fasting.

Therefore, you are essentially limited to three beverages:

- Water or mineral water
- Unsweetened tea
- Black coffee

However, drinks like green tea or black coffee still contain about 2.5 calories per cup. Nonetheless, most experts agree that this amount does not interrupt fat burning (ketosis) and is therefore negligible.

In addition to ketosis, a second mechanism is responsible for the lion's share of fasting's health benefits – autophagy.[224]

As has already been explained, our cells' recycling system is deactivated by consuming any of the three macronutrients.

Therefore, the simplistic approach that any caloric food breaks a fast was born.

We will see that this approach is not entirely correct when we look at the disadvantages of dirty intermittent fasting. That is why, for example, in clean fasting, non-nutritive sweeteners such as stevia are not allowed.

Moreover, there still exists an increase in clean fasting – autophagy fasting. Proponents of pure autophagy fasting consume only water and sometimes natural salt such as pink Himalayan salt.

However, this is not so much an intermittent fasting method as a therapeutic fasting method. Therefore, salt is allowed as well. Because the body loses sodium over several days of fasting, this can cause dizziness and headaches.

Dirty Intermittent Fasting

Dirty or lazy intermittent fasting is a new term that allows food intake of up to 100 calories during fasting.

For example, dirty intermittent fasting allows the following foods and sweeteners (in beverages) during the 16 hours:

- **2 tbsp. cream:** 30 calories / 0.8 g carbohydrate / 0.6 g protein / 11.0 g fat.[225]

- **2 tbsp. whole milk:** 18.3 calories / 1.6 g carbohydrates / 1.0 g protein / 1.0 g fat.[226]

- **2 tbsp. almond milk:** 5 calories / 0.2 g carbohydrates / 0.1 g protein / 0.4 g fat.[227]

- **14 grams grass-fed butter:** 100 calories / 0.0 g carbohydrates / 0.0 g protein / 11.4 g fat.[228]

- **2 tsp. MCT oil:** 84 calories / 0.0 g carbohydrates / 0.0 g protein / 10 g fat.[229]

- **1 cup bone broth:** 100 calories / 1.5 g carbohydrates / 0.9 g protein / 0.4 g fat.[230]

- **1 lemon (juice squeezed):** 11.7 calories / 4.1 g carbohydrates / 0.2 g protein / 0.0 g fat.[231]

- **1 can coke zero:** 0.0 calories / 0.0 g carbohydrates / 0.0 g protein / 0.0 g fat.[232]

- **1 pack splenda (sucralose):** 3.4 calories / 0.9 g carbohydrates / 0.0 g protein / 0.0 g fat.[233]

- **1 pack stevia (pure):** 0.0 calories / 0.0 g carbohydrates / 0.0 g protein / 0.0 g fat.[234]

- **1 tbsp. agave syrup:** 60 calories / 21.3 g carbohydrates / 0.0 g protein / 0.0 g fat.[235]

- **1 tbsp. honey:** 64 calories / 17.3 g carbohydrates / 0.1 g protein / 0.0 g fat.[236]

- **1 sugar-free chewing gum:** 5.4 calories / 1.9 g carbohydrates / 0.0 g protein / 0.0 g fat.[237]

In summary, dirty intermittent fasting allows diet drinks, sweeteners, and other additions to tea and coffee, while not exceeding 100 calories.

Diet sodas, low-calorie sweeteners, and some food sound like a relaxed version of intermittent fasting.

Can this lazy approach to intermittent fasting be similarly practical as the clean one?

Is Dirty Fasting Effective?

Dirty fasting has only one rule, limiting energy intake to 100 calories during fasting. But that's where the problem lies.

Technically, any macronutrient breaks the fast in terms of autophagy.

However, experts overwhelmingly agree that minimal amounts, such as in green tea, cannot significantly interfere with autophagy.

Nevertheless, consuming 100 calories will reduce autophagy to an absolute baseline level. Hence, this calorie intake eliminates most rejuvenating effects of fasting.

But when it comes to weight loss, the three macronutrients can by no means be lumped together since the storage hormone insulin regulates our body weight.

While pure fat such as butter does not elevate insulin, a tablespoon of honey spikes blood glucose and insulin levels.

Similarly, protein without the protective effect of fat can stimulate insulin secretion. Thus, protein powder in coffee, for example, is not a good idea.[238]

Although many nutritionists reduce foods to their effects on blood glucose, this approach is doomed to failure.

It ignores that it is not only blood glucose that can cause an insulin response.

For example, the following zero-calorie sweeteners can also stimulate insulin secretion:[239,240,241,242,243]

- Acesulfame-K (zero drinks)
- Aspartame (diet soda)
- Sucralose (Splenda)
- Stevia
- Monk fruit

Since dirty fasting completely ignores the insulin perspective, it breaks fasting and ketosis. Therefore, it cannot be as effective as clean intermittent fasting.

Which Approach Is Better?

In contrast to clean intermittent fasting, the disadvantages outweigh the advantages of dirty fasting. Especially since dirty intermittent fasting only relates to calories and not insulin levels, it is not nearly as effective for weight loss.

However, dirty fasting can work if we modify the essential rule to include insulin in our considerations.

In this case, the allowed calorie intake during the fasting period is limited to pure fat, which does not stimulate insulin secretion.

As a result, we get so-called fat fasting. For example, this legitimizes the ever-popular Bulletproof Coffee since only butter, ghee, coconut, or MCT oil are in it.

Due to consistently low insulin levels, many achieve excellent weight loss despite consuming pure fat coffee or tea drinks.

In addition, fatty drinks help satiate beginners to last longer when fasting.

For this reason, combining a ketogenic diet and intermittent fasting is most effective for weight loss.

How Dirty Fasting Can Work

The dirty intermittent fasting approach is ineffective because it restricts foods to calorie values.

If you still have trouble fasting for an extended time, I suggest a dirty fat fasting approach that evaluates foods based on insulin response.

Our examples of beverage additions result in a yes and no list for effective dirty fasting.

Accordingly, the following foods are allowed in dirty fat fasting:

- **2 tbsp. cream:** 30 calories / 0.8 g carbohydrate / 0.6 g protein / 11.0 g fat.[244]

- **14 grams grass-fed butter:** 100 calories / 0.0 g carbs / 0.0 g protein / 11.4 g fat.[245]

- **2 tsp. MCT oil:** 84 calories / 0.0 g carbohydrates / 0.0 g protein / 10 g fat.[246]

- **1 cup bone broth:** 100 calories / 1.5 g carbohydrate / 0.9 g protein / 0.4 g fat.[247]

Although fat interferes with autophagy, it does not stop fat burning.

In contrast, the following foods will affect your weight loss success:

- **2 tbsp. whole milk:** 18.3 calories / 1.6 g carbohydrates / 1.0 g protein / 1.0 g fat.[248]

- **1 can coke zero:** 0.0 calories / 0.0 g carbohydrates / 0.0 g protein / 0.0 g fat.[249]

- **1 pack splenda (sucralose):** 3.4 calories / 0.9 g carbohydrates / 0.0 g protein / 0.0 g fat.[250]

- **1 pack stevia (pure):** 0.0 calories / 0.0 g carbohydrates / 0.0 g protein / 0.0 g fat.[251]

- **1 tbsp. agave syrup:** 60 calories / 21.3 g carbohydrates / 0.0 g protein / 0.0 g fat.[252]

- **1 tbsp. honey:** 64 calories / 17.3 g carbohydrates / 0.1 g protein / 0.0 g fat.[253]

In addition, non-nutritive sweeteners fuel cravings, according to science.[254]

The subtleties of dirty fasting introduce the following essential point when successfully integrating intermittent fasting 16/8 into your daily work routine.

Top 5 Intermittent Fasting Mistakes

Every person goes through a learning process at the beginning of a new routine. The journey includes making mistakes because only from these can be learned.

Nevertheless, I want to save you time at this point and explain five common mistakes that intermittent fasting beginners usually make entirely unconsciously.

1. Milk in Your Coffee

We have already addressed the most common mistake in my experience, especially since drinking is where most errors occur during fasting.

When drinking water, coffee, or tea, unintended mistakes repeatedly happen during intermittent fasting. But in most cases, people usually only lack reliable information.

Thus, many fasting beginners get carried away, perhaps adding a splash of milk or a packet of sugar to their coffee.

But these subtle little things can have significant effects. By raising blood sugar and insulin levels, they break the fast. So, time and time again, a good portion of the health benefits and, more importantly, the progress in losing weight are negated.

For example, ketogenic diet followers tend to forget that a so-called Bulletproof Coffee also breaks the fast.

So butter, coconut, or MCT oil in the coffee helps against hunger in between but prevents the full health effect of fasting.

Although bone broth is a prime source of electrolytes and fat, it too technically breaks the fast and should only be used as a jump start. Once you get used to intermittent fasting, it is taboo or no longer necessary, just like Bulletproof Coffee.

Moreover, many people don't know that while diet soda is sugar-free, that doesn't automatically mean it can't break a fast, as already discussed.

2. Too Little Salt

Apart from fat, hardly anything has been demonized as much as salt for decades. Not only advertising campaigns but also doctors have caused this distorted image. Nevertheless, salt is not as bad as its reputation.

Few people are aware that we cannot survive without salt. Although a daily requirement of two grams is currently recommended, our ancestors instinctively consumed 2-3 times as much salt.

Amazingly, even today, the countries with the highest salt consumption have the lowest rates of cardiovascular disease.

One example is South Korea, where sodium consumption is exceptionally high due to the popularity of kimchi - fermented Chinese cabbage with plenty of salt.[255]

Recent studies increasingly show that it is not excess salt but deficiency of potassium that causes hypertension.[256]

And potassium deficiency is again part of our essential lifestyle. The higher the degree of processing of foods, the less natural potassium they contain on average.

In addition, salt is the natural antagonist of sugar, takes the bitter taste out of our food, and works against cravings.

Unlike sugar, salt has a negative feedback loop. When your body has had enough salt, you don't crave it anymore.

For example, I have trouble eating salty soup. With cake and sugar, however, things are different. Sound familiar?

Moreover, recent studies suggest that too little salt intake may be more harmful to our health than the other way around.

Accordingly, endocrinologist and fasting pioneer, Dr. Jason Fung, reports that physical side effects of fasting are usually due to too little salt consumption.

For example, he says, these are especially headaches and dizziness.[257]

Furthermore, he has observed in his diabetes clinic that salt intake is essential for weight loss, especially in women. In this context, we must also note that salt can help prevent type 2 diabetes.6

While sugar consumption promotes insulin resistance and body fat storage, salt increases insulin sensitivity and helps you lose weight instead.[258]

Good options for getting healthy salt into your diet include pink Himalayan salt or Celtic sea salt. Since these salts usually don't contain chemical additives like anti-caking agents, they are more natural.

Nevertheless, as with any other dietary change, it is essential to consult with your trusted physician.

People suffering from chronic kidney disease or certain cardiovascular diseases must watch their sodium intake.

If you experience headaches while fasting, the following home remedies can help:

- **Salt to taste:** Listen to your body and dare to salt food properly when it asks for it.

- **Drink bone broth:** Many fasting beginners find it helpful to drink bone broth or unsweetened pickle juice until the body gets used to the lifestyle.

- **Use sole water:** If you don't have sugar-free pickle juice or bone broth on hand, dissolve a pinch of salt in a glass of water — the same works with tea or coffee.

- **Cut back on carbohydrates:** Carbohydrates retain water in the body. If you eat bread, cookies, protein, or granola bars between fasts, water will be stored and flushed out with sodium, causing headaches afterward.

3. Poor Diet

Although beginners are often afraid of not getting enough nutrients during intermittent fasting, in my experience, this is somewhat unjustified.

During fasting, the hormone system sets the course for fat burning. However, this does not mean you have to eat less. Instead, you get your nutrients more concentrated in two larger meals.

Nevertheless, you are still responsible for the quality of the food you eat.

Although intermittent fasting basically works with any diet, you can do much wrong and counteract health progress.

If you have just started intermittent fasting, your body flushes excess water and electrolytes through the gastrointestinal tract.

But that is nothing to worry about and can also have several other triggers, such as excessive caffeine consumption from tea or coffee.

Hence, you must ensure essential electrolytes such as potassium, magnesium, and sodium throughout your diet.

Nonetheless, intermittent fasting will not cause diarrhea in the long run.

Instead, you are likely to get diarrhea if you break the fast. But that is a natural reaction when the gastrointestinal tract starts working again after an extended fasting period.

However, if this condition persists for an extended time with a consistent fasting window, it's much more likely that you're simply eating poorly.

Many people's intestines struggle with the following usual suspects:

- Refined carbohydrates
- Legumes high in fiber and lectins
- Too much dairy (lactose and beta-casein A1)

Those who base their fasting diet on baking goods, sweets, beans, and low-fat dairy products could cause noticeable complications. In addition, you will hardly lose weight with such a diet.

In addition to one extreme of diarrhea, the other extreme of constipation can occur due to a fiber-rich diet.

Since fiber is that part of plant food that the body cannot digest, it increases stool volume.

And as researchers have now correctly recognized, it isn't easy to pass large volumes through a narrow opening.

Nonetheless, some people believe they can prevent constipation by increasing fiber intake.

But studies show that the exact opposite is true.[259]

In addition to reducing the above foods, the following beverages can help you with digestive problems:

- **Water:** Increased water consumption is always welcome and necessary to prevent dehydration.

- **Bone broth:** When diarrhea sufferers, increased electrolyte intake through drinks such as bone broth, pickle juice, or sole water is essential.

- **Other drinks:** Avoid sugary, caffeinated, and diet soda.

4. Inadequate Hydration

A common mistake in intermittent fasting is that people like to confuse thirst with hunger.

Instead of reaching for water or tea, we go for a protein bar since solid food also provides fluid to a certain degree.

However, when we forgo familiar snacks, we often don't replenish the fluids they gave us.

As a result, we think we feel hungry. Accordingly, during periods of fasting and between meals, you often don't crave food but simply a craving for fluid that needs to be satisfied.

Accordingly, some people need regular reminders in their daily lives to take in enough fluids.

So how much do you need to drink during a fasting period?

Fluid intake during intermittent fasting cannot be generalized.

Neither do utopian recommendations of 5 liters of water per day apply to everyone, nor can you calculate fluid needs based on weight, height, and age.

Moreover, overhydration is just as harmful as dehydration. Nevertheless, a simple rule of thumb applies: drink when you are thirsty.

As is often the case, it is better to listen to your body. You don't have to force yourself constantly to drink if you're not thirsty. The same should apply to everyday life.

When in doubt, a glass of water or tea won't hurt. With more extended periods of fasting and experience, you will get a better sense of when you are thirsty.

The following options are available to counteract any hunger pangs you may feel in between meals:

- **Mineral water:** The carbonic acid in mineral water helps alleviate hunger pangs. Moreover, it replenishes electrolytes your body loses through urine.

- **A glass of water:** Drink a cup of tea or a glass of water when you feel hungry and wait 30 minutes. If hunger subsides, you are just thirsty.

- **Reminders:** If you have trouble drinking enough fluids, use your cell phone alarm clock for regular reminders.

5. Lack of Activity

A persistent myth about fasting is that you must always take it easy, especially if you feel tired.

If you already feel tired, the surest way to eventually feel terrible is to rest even more. Instead, activity can help the body go fat-burning more efficiently.

After our bodies try to conserve energy where they can, fat-burning often requires physical activity to get it going.

If you feel fatigued while fasting, it's often a sign that carbohydrate stores are depleting. However, we can't burn fat until these short-term batteries are empty.

Then the human body tells us with sluggishness that quickly available energy is running low. However, it does not want to expend additional metabolic energy to burn body fat immediately.

Accordingly, body fat is like a saving account only tackled when the checking account (our carbohydrate stores in the liver and skeletal muscles) is empty.[260]

That's why it helps to increase your energy needs with exercise. This way, you force your body to switch to burning body fat.

Another mistake is to overdo it with an intense workout. On the other hand, a leisurely walk or even yoga will help to boost fat burning.

Nonetheless, it is crucial to listen to your body when fasting. If you feel good with fasting and weight lifting, go for it.

However, since fasting doesn't run away, you can always break your fast when you feel uncomfortable doing it.

For me, strength training and intermittent fasting work very well together. This way, an exceptionally high amount of growth hormone is released, which in turn helps to build muscles more efficiently.

It is different regarding intensive endurance training, such as marathon preparation. In my experience, the body's increased appetite and need for recovery speak against more extended periods of fasting.

As long as you feel sluggish, however, the following tips can help you:

- **Exercise:** Don't stop moving altogether if you feel low on energy. Otherwise, you'll become even more sluggish. So grab the bike or take the dog for a walk.

- **Activity:** Treat the fasting day or period like any other. Although fasting beginners are usually nervous, it's no big deal. Nature designed our bodies for it. Housework or gardening can distract you and keep you active.

- **Measure:** If you have a fatigue attack, a 15-minute walk can help.

Intermittent Fasting and Working Out

Intermittent fasting doesn't require you to take it easy all the time. On the contrary, the fasted state improves the health benefits of exercise.

Furthermore, intermittent fasting can help you build muscle if you use it correctly. Here you can find out how to combine it perfectly.

Can You Workout While Fasting?

A persistent myth about fasting is that you must always take it easy. If you already feel tired, the surest way to eventually feel terrible is to rest even more.

Instead, an activity can help your body kick into gear and get more efficient at burning fat.

For this reason, whether it makes sense to exercise during intermittent fasting can usually only be answered in the affirmative.

Also, fasted exercise amplifies its benefits. If you feel just great while fasting, you must, therefore, by no means lie around like a couch potato.

Working out and intermittent fasting also promote blood sugar regulation and can prevent even rare digestion problems during fasting.

Nevertheless, especially if you are new to intermittent fasting, you should start with mild physical activity and always listen to your body.

However, you do not need to work out to lose weight with intermittent fasting.

Can You Lose Weight Without Exercising?

In principle, intermittent fasting can work without exercise since it sets the hormonal course for weight loss and improved health.

Ultimately, obesity is more a hormonal imbalance than a caloric one, as the world-renowned neuroendocrinologist Dr. Robert Lustig concludes.[261]

Insulin, the storage hormone in our body, is the key to this process.

Those unhealthily high insulin levels that plague us today have two primary causes:

- High-carbohydrate diets
- Constant eating

Intermittent fasting addresses the latter problem by restoring a natural balance between eating and fasting.

To finally burn stored body fat as a source of energy, the carbohydrate stores in the liver and muscle mass must first be emptied.

In addition to intermittent fasting, working out also helps to do so. Accordingly, sport increases the energy demand during intermittent fasting, which causes the glycogen stores to deplete even faster.

That is why sport in a fasted state can significantly accelerate fat burning. Those who do not eat for a long time and practice sports on an empty stomach thus increase fat-burning effectiveness.

Nevertheless, intermittent fasting can work even without exercise, as long as you do not constantly fill the carbohydrate stores.

Therefore, combining intermittent fasting with a low-carbohydrate diet like the keto diet is beneficial.

Moreover, you must know that exercise triggers a compensatory effect and increases appetite.[262]

For this reason, what you eat after exercise is even more critical for successful weight loss.

When Should You Work Out?

As we have already concluded, exercise during intermittent fasting makes sense just within the fasting period.

So whether you exercise in the morning or the evening is not significant. What is more important is that you have fasted for a sufficient time. The longer the fasting period before exercise, the greater the effect on fat oxidation.

Therefore, the best time for exercise depends on your intermittent fasting plan. If you skip breakfast due to 16/8, a workout before lunch will have the most excellent effect.

If, instead, you fast for 24 hours from dinner to dinner, exercise is best in the evening before the meal.

Benefits of Fasting and Working Out

Exercise and fasting can help you reach your health goals faster, especially if they involve fat loss. Here are some of the most important benefits of working out in a fasted state.

1. Enhanced Fat Burning

Combining working out and intermittent fasting is especially smart if you want to improve your body composition.

When carbohydrate stores are empty due to fasting, the body sustainably taps into fat tissue as the next available energy source.[263]

In contrast, eating carbohydrates before working out inhibits potential fat burning.[264]

Therefore, the combination with a low-carbohydrate or ketogenic diet is even more efficient because the glycogen stores are already empty in this case. Thus, the body can immediately start fat oxidation.

Along these lines, studies on fasted exercise show that you burn more fat this way and the amount of fat released per cell also increases.[265]

Moreover, further studies suggest that more blood flows to the abdominal area when fasted, helping burn fat cells stored in this area.[266]

2. Increased Autophagy

Besides fat burning, autophagy is the main benefit of fasting.

And fasting is one of the best ways to activate autophagy.[267]

The intercellular recycling system kicks into high gear when you don't eat for about 14 hours.[268]

In addition to fasting, regular and intense exercise can also really kick-start the process.

Accordingly, one study discovered increased autophagy markers in people who played soccer all their lives. In a direct comparison, people of the same age who had not exercised their entire lives performed significantly worse.[269]

Also, scientists could detect autophagy activity in the liver, muscle, pancreas, and adipose tissue in mice regularly exercising on a treadmill.[270]

Moreover, according to a recent study, exercise intensity is more crucial for autophagy in muscle cells than the fasting state itself.[271]

Hence, *High-Intensity Interval Training (HIIT)* is an excellent way to achieve autophagy incredibly quickly in combination with fasting.

3. Improved Muscle Gains

Fasting is one of the most effective ways to stimulate the *human growth hormone (HGH)*.[272]

Hence it helps promote bone, cartilage, and muscle development. As a result, you get more substantial muscles and protection against age-related bone and muscle loss.

By fasting, you maximize the release of growth hormone until you break the fasting window after exercising with a meal. This way, you send the body into an anabolic state at the right time for targeted muscle building.

Since the production of growth hormone decreases after 30, you can use intermittent fasting to help your body continue to produce this vital neurotransmitter.

Accordingly, HGH helps with muscle recovery after exercise and sets the stage for healthy bones, organs, and longevity.[273]

But again, it is low insulin levels that enable growth hormone release. Regular intermittents of fasting, such as the 16/8 method, create the foundation for this.

4. Enhanced Endurance

When you practice cardio exercise, your endurance is only as good as your body's ability to deliver necessary oxygen to target cells.

Endurance training can help increase this process of oxygen delivery. The measure of this is the maximal oxygen uptake, often referred to as VO2-Max.

VO2-Max measures the maximum amount of oxygen your body uses per minute during an endurance workout when you're pushing yourself hard.

Increasing this value allows your body to take in more oxygen and deliver it to your muscles. This way, you can improve your performance during cardio workouts.

One study compared the VO2-Max values of people in a fasted and fed state. The group that had cereal for breakfast performed significantly worse than those who ate nothing after getting up.

At the start of the study, all participants had average VO2-Max values of about 3.5 liters per minute (L/min). After ergometer training, the fasted group's VO2 max increased by about 10 percent.

In contrast, the fed group saw only a 2.5 percent improvement in VO2 max.[274]

In short, intermittent fasting allows people to increase their maximal oxygen uptake through exercise significantly better than those who eat breakfast or eat before a workout.

5. Fewer Digestion Issues

Have you ever experienced indigestion or nausea after eating a pre-workout protein bar or shake?

If so, you're not alone in this. These pre-workouts have become mainstream in the fitness and food industries because they have good money to make.

However, as we learned before, pre-workout food hinders performance enhancement rather than the other way round. Moreover, bars and shakes are full of carbohydrates and proteins that increase insulin secretion.

For this reason, they ultimately prevent fat burning as well.

Therefore, exercising during intermittent fasting helps you avoid digestive discomfort and ensures you reach your goals faster.

How to Combine Exercise and Fasting

Combining working out and intermittent fasting can generate sensational results. But if you want to succeed, there are three basic rules.

1. Listen to Your Body

Common sense is always needed when doing sports. With this in mind, you should regulate your training intensity based on your overall feeling, especially if you have just started intermittent fasting.

If you don't feel well, refrain from the training session and take a day off.

Unless you're just feeling sluggish, grab a bike or go for a walk. Don't hesitate to hit the gym if you feel fit while fasting.

For example, after I get up, yoga helps me generate extra energy and a sense of mindfulness for the whole day.

2. Do Not Eat Before Working Out

Authors often overlook this vital point, mostly when they are selling sports nutrition.

If you drink an energy drink or eat protein bars before exercise, the carbohydrates in them inhibit fat burning.[275]

Since the increased insulin level blocks the enzyme responsible for fat breakdown, this is hardly surprising.[276]

Moreover, the body then preferentially consumes the energy supplied by food in the bloodstream.

The need to supply the body with external energy before training is a widespread misconception drilled into us by advertising campaigns for decades.

In the end, it would be far more effective to burn stored body fat instead.

Therefore, there are only two real reasons to eat before exercise:

- You want to build body fat in addition to muscle mass
- You are a professional athlete and train three times a day

For this reason, the ubiquitous orientation from hobby sports to competitive sports has prevented countless people from getting into the shape they crave.

3. Stay Hydrated

Whether in a fasted state or not, you need to be adequately hydrated to get a top-notch workout.

We do not absorb the fluids we usually get from foods when we fast. Therefore, it is crucial to ensure adequate hydration before and after exercise.

Drinking water just before training is not enough. After all, it takes a while for the water to get from the stomach to the muscles.

For this reason, it makes sense to drink enough water at least 30 minutes before training and not just immediately before.

If you drink sufficient fluids before and after your workout, you should not feel cravings afterward. These cravings usually occur because we are dehydrated.

For example, this way, you'll find it easier to work out in the morning and not break your fast until noon.

The increased release of adrenaline during intermittent fasting helps many people work out more consistently.

On top of that, it boosts fat burning.[277]

Besides, working out and intermittent fasting help reduce stress and cope with anxiety.

In my experience, fasting also makes you go into workouts more vigor and helps you concentrate better.

Furthermore, exercise also boosts ketosis, which in turn increases the positive effect.

The bottom line, therefore, is that a low-carbohydrate diet like the keto diet is, in my experience, the best way to maximize the health benefits of intermittent fasting.

How to Fight Cravings Naturally

Even though science is still far from being able to fully explain all the hormones surrounding hunger and their complex interplay, tips can be derived for sustainable satiety.

We cannot completely control our appetite, but we can bring our modern lifestyle and thus our hormone balance back into the equilibrium that nature originally intended.

Controlling Hunger Hormones

Ghrelin is the essential circulating hunger hormone in the body, closely related to NPY, the primary hunger hormone in the central nervous system.

Together they initiate hunger while being influenced by other peripheral hormones.

Although ghrelin stimulates appetite, you should by no means consider taking ghrelin blockers. Ghrelin is also vital for learning, memory, gastric acid secretion, sleep-wake cycles, and reward behavior and should not be artificially unbalanced.[279]

Instead, studies show that the eating behavior itself can curb the release of hunger hormones.

1. Focus Protein-Rich Foods

According to an Oxford study that compared the consumption of a high-protein meal with a high-carbohydrate meal, protein consumption can significantly lower ghrelin levels in the body.[280]

Similarly, in Oxford, researchers found that reducing protein in the diet caused a more significant release of NPY and more body fat.[281]

2. Increase Intake of Healthy Fats

High levels of NPY fuel cravings for carbohydrates. In contrast, fat consumption inhibits NPY activity more than other macronutrients, which curbs cravings.[282]

To summarize, natural foods high in fat and protein are excellent choices to curb appetite.

In addition to fattier cuts of meat, fatty fish, such as salmon or mackerel, is ideal, as its omega-3 fatty acids can further support satiety.[283]

3 Avoid Fructose

The supposed fruit sugar is often marketed as healthy, which it is not. Fructose is the sweet molecule besides glucose in conventional table sugar. Therefore, a piece of dextrose (glucose) is not distinctively sweet because it lacks fructose.

Metabolic researchers have found that diets high in fructose can increase ghrelin levels, causing obesity.[284]

Accordingly, the sweet molecule fuels cravings and promotes changes in the brain's reward system, leading to overconsumption.

In addition, fructose causes the development of new fat and insulin resistance in the liver, leading to chronic metabolic diseases such as fatty liver and type 2 diabetes.

These effects on the liver become easier to understand when we realize that fructose is closely related to alcohol and can cause the same diseases.

The fermentation of fructose produces ethanol – alcohol. The main difference is that fructose is 100% metabolized in the liver and not in the brain, sparing sensations of intoxication and hangovers.[285]

In addition, fructose significantly affects the satiety hormone leptin, as we will see shortly.

Increasing Satiety Hormones

Sustained satiety goes far beyond a short-term feeling of fullness due to stomach distension. Since the essential satiety hormones have been more adequately researched, we can draw meaningful conclusions about which meals make us feel full in the long term and which do not.

Interesting starting points also exist regarding the influences of other lifestyle factors such as exercise and sleep on our satiety hormones. According to science, here are the best tips to increase those hormones that cause satiety.

1. Reduce Carbs

This first point may sound like old news, yet it cannot be repeated often enough. The industrialization of food production has creepily, yet significantly, increased carbohydrate consumption over the decades.

Refined carbohydrates like sugar can turn off the leptin receptors in the brain, so you need longer or higher levels of leptin to get full.[286]

To summarize, added sugar in foods makes you hungry for more.

In this regard, the fructose in sugar is more dangerous than other carbohydrates in developing leptin resistance and obesity.[287]

Therefore, it is advisable to avoid high fructose concentrations such as in high-fructose corn syrup, agave syrup, candy, and other processed foods.

Moreover, carbohydrate-rich meals stimulate the satiety hormone PYY the least, and their level decreases rapidly afterward. In contrast, PYY continues to rise for hours after high-fat and high-protein meals.[288]

For this reason, processed carbohydrates such as those in cookies or other baking goods do not keep you full for long. Moreover, they promote inflammation in the body.[289]

And inflammation is often associated with obesity and inhibits the release of GLP-1, thereby inhibiting satiety.[290]

2. Prefer Natural Fats to Seed Oils

Refined seed oils, such as soybean, sunflower, or canola oil, are just as pro-inflammatory as refined carbohydrates.[291]

And like sugars, they are found in a wide variety of highly processed foods today.

In contrast, extra virgin olive oil could increase GLP-1 levels.[292]

Furthermore, consumption of natural fats in extra virgin olive oil, grass-fed butter, or grass-fed beef supports CCK production, thereby maintaining satiety longer.[293]

Although fat is more nutritious than carbohydrates, excessive fat consumption does not lead to leptin resistance.[294]

Moreover, the secretion of the satiety hormone PYY increases proportionally to the amount of fat consumed via diet.[295]

In short, a high-fat, low-carbohydrate diet such as the keto diet is ideal for increasing satiety and avoiding cravings.

3. Eat Enough Protein

Like healthy fats, protein increases the release of satiety hormones in the gut.

Accordingly, one study found that a high-protein diet, as opposed to a high-carbohydrate diet, can help increase CCK levels and thus feelings of satiety.[296]

Similarly, protein-rich foods can increase GLP-1 levels.[297] In particular, collagen, the essential protein for skin, hair, bone, and joints, promotes satiety via GLP-1.[298]

Regarding PYY, high-protein meals satiate even more effectively than high-fat meals.[299]

4. Get Regular, Quality Sleep

Here is the evidence if you've ever heard that sleep is vital for weight loss.

Among many other essential tasks, sleep helps you use leptin properly. Researchers have found that shorter sleep results in lower levels of the satiety hormone leptin in the body.[300]

A brand new study even states that sleep deprivation can lead to obesity and subsequently type 2 diabetes by impairing leptin regulation, as it increases appetite and food intake.[301]

Furthermore, studies consistently show that sleep deprivation leads to increased ghrelin levels and decreased leptin.[302]

A recent review of 21 studies involving 2,250 individuals concluded that reduced sleep duration is associated with increased ghrelin levels, whereas sleep disturbance affects leptin and ghrelin levels.[303]

Consequently, sleep hygiene significantly affects the regulation of appetite. To avoid the risk of increasing your body mass index, you should regularly get more than 7 hours of quality net sleep per night.[304]

5. Don't Rely on Exercise Alone

Exercise helps increase leptin sensitivity, increasing the hormone's perception and satiety.[305]

However, overall, study results are mixed regarding the effects of exercise on hunger and satiety hormones.

While individuals of average weight can increase their PYY levels with exercise, overweight individuals achieved this result only with long-term training for at least 32 weeks.[306]

In contrast, there is evidence that high-intensity interval training (HIIT) or the combination of aerobic and strength training could increase CCK levels.[307]

On the other hand, intense training could not affect NPY levels to the extent that weight loss could result.[308,309]

However, do not forget that exercise promotes hunger. And for some people, this compensatory effect of food intake is even more significant than it should be.[310]

Accordingly, exercise is not the tool of choice for regulating appetite. If the necessary dietary intervention is not provided, athletic ambitions can backfire by craving foods that reduce satiety, promoting overeating in the long run.

To summarize, Hunger is not a bad feeling per se. Instead, hunger and satiety are standard physiological signals that keep us alive and contribute to the body's optimal functioning.

Our lifestyle, marked by psychological stress and changes in food production, affects the natural balance of hunger and satiety hormones.

Although appetite and its hormones represent a complex interplay that we do not yet understand precisely, research has yielded results in recent years.

Highly processed foods with refined carbohydrates and added sugars make us more hungry in the long run.

In particular, the fructose in sugar inhibits satiety signals and fuels cravings.[311]

In contrast to these processed carbohydrates, natural fatty acids and proteins can contribute to lasting satiety and lower inflammation levels.

As a result, we get a low-carbohydrate, high-fat diet that relies on natural protein sources such as fatty fish.

Accordingly, brand-new studies highlight that such ketogenic diets prevent an increase in the hunger hormone ghrelin, which is otherwise seen after weight loss, and instead reduce feelings of hunger.[312]

In a direct comparison with a *low-fat, high-carbohydrate (LFHC)* diet, a *low-carb, high-fat (LCHF)* diet significantly increased satiety after it released 55% more PYY in the gut.[313]

In addition to diet, sleep is the second major factor that can help curb appetite via healthy hormone balance. Therefore, you should always prioritize regular, quality sleep.

Intermittent fasting can help to do so.

In one study, female subjects could noticeably improve sleep quality, REM sleep, and balance after only two weeks of intermittent fasting.

In addition, they were able to improve their performance during the day.[314]

Diet for a Healthy Cycle

Besides stress reduction, nutrition is the essential lifestyle factor that can regulate hormone balance and reduce inflammation in the body.

For this reason, you will find the best and worst foods for PMS. On top of that, based on recent studies, I have elicited why some diets may be beneficial in alleviating PMS symptoms.

Best Food Choices

A woman's menstrual cycle and its impact on premenstrual syndrome are characterized by fluctuating estrogen and progesterone levels.

Therefore, below you will find the best natural foods to relieve PMS symptoms depending on the cycle phase.

Based on this, you can optimize your diet throughout the month.

Follicular Phase

The first main phase of the cycle is divided into menstrual and proliferation phases. Below, you will find the best foods to regulate these menstrual cycle phases naturally.

Menstrual Phase

The first days of the female cycle are characterized by menstruation. During this time, there is an additional need for the following micronutrients:

- Iron
- Omega-3 fatty acids
- Magnesium

While magnesium has been shown to help with PMS symptoms such as cravings, depression, and anxiety,[315] marine omega-3 fatty acids relieve period cramps more effectively than ibuprofen.[316]

Last but not least, iron is useful. Since women excrete an average of half a liter of iron per year during menstruation, they are more likely to suffer from iron deficiency than men.[317]

The bottom line is a selection of foods that can supply all three micronutrients in excellent balance:

- Mussels[318]
- Salmon[319]
- Offal such as liver[320]
- Beef[321]
- Walnuts[322]

Salmon and beef are proper foods during the early menstrual cycle phases

Proliferation Phase

During the second stage of the follicular phase, estrogen levels increase. And it is a sensitive issue.

In addition to the menstrual cycle, it regulates female curves, fat distribution, mood, and in some cases, even memory function.[323,324]

Therefore, unbalanced estrogen levels can lead to depression, insomnia, or brain fog.

Accordingly, you should ensure that your estrogen levels remain balanced during the proliferation phase. Fortunately, diet is one of the most effective ways to regulate estrogen levels.

When it comes to healthy estrogen levels, one all-rounder combines all the positive effects: Cruciferous vegetables. These include, in particular:

- Cauliflower
- Broccoli
- Kale
- Cabbage
- Brussels sprouts

These vegetables contain as many as three active compounds that can naturally regulate estrogen levels:

- **Indole-3-Carbinol (I3C):** These plant compounds can help remove excess estrogen from the body. Studies suggest that cruciferous vegetables may protect against hormone-dependent cancers such as breast cancer in women.[325]

- **Dietary fiber:** Although cabbage vegetables are generally low in carbohydrates, they are rich in dietary fiber, which helps lower estrogen levels while progesterone levels remain.[326]

- **Phytoestrogens:** Cruciferous vegetables' lignans block estrogen action in tissues, increasing SHBG and regulating estrogen levels. In addition, the antiestrogenic effects may help reduce the risk of hormone-related cancers, such as breast, uterine, or ovarian.[327]

Other good sources of these phytoestrogens are flaxseeds and berries.

Moreover, polyphenol-containing beverages such as green tea, red wine, and even coffee provide lignans beneficial during the proliferation phase.

Ovulation

While some women do not notice their ovulation, others already experience PMS symptoms. These include, in particular, cravings, breast pain, or bloating during ovulation.[328]

Fortunately, these early signs of premenstrual syndrome can also be alleviated with the right foods. In this regard, the following nutrients are crucial:

- Proteins
- Healthy fats
- Vitamin B6

Whole foods with a large load of proteins and healthy fats are the first choice to stimulate the release of the satiety hormones cholecystokinin, peptide YY, GLP-1, or leptin.[329]

Low leptin levels, high sugar, and other carbohydrate consumption usually cause PMS-related cravings.[330]

If you experience PMS symptoms around ovulation, which may be due to water retention, vitamin B6 is that micronutrient that can help you.[331]

In addition to bloating and abdominal discomfort, vitamin B6 can help with breast pain and tenderness.[332]

In summary, a few foods again stand out as being able to both fight cravings and maximize vitamin B6 intake:

- Salmon[333]
- Eggs[334]
- Chicken liver[335]
- Beef[336]
- Pistachios[337]

Besides the numerous animal foods, pistachios are an excellent vegan option for early PMS symptoms. On the one hand, they are rich in healthy fats and proteins, and on the other hand, just one cup of pistachios can provide the entire daily requirement of vitamin B6.[338]

Luteal Phase

Cramps, mood swings, depression, insomnia, or headaches are more common during the luteal phase.

You can prevent the full range of PMS symptoms by additionally incorporating the following foods:

- Magnesium
- Anti-inflammatory foods

Researchers found elevated inflammatory markers in 20 women who suffered from premenstrual syndrome, particularly in the luteal phase.[339]

Moreover, other studies show that women struggling with PMS symptoms often have low magnesium levels.[340]

For this reason, some women may crave chocolate (cocoa) before the menstrual phase. These cravings are often less about satisfying a sweet tooth than about the mood-regulating effect of magnesium.

Research shows that women who take magnesium and vitamin B6 experience less premenstrual depression, anxiety, and cravings.[341]

Because they contain magnesium, protein, healthy fats, and other anti-inflammatory nutrients, the following foods are ideal companions to combat cravings and all PMS symptoms during the luteal phase:

- Mussels[342]
- Halibut[343]
- Salmon[344]
- Cocoa nibs[345]
- Almonds[346]
- Pistachios[347]
- Walnuts[348]

Fatty fish and seafood are at the top of this list for a good reason. Their omega-3 fatty acids are not only anti-inflammatory but also more effective against period cramps than common medications.[349]

While nuts have fewer anti-inflammatory proper-ties than fatty fish, they impress with magnesium, vitamin B6, and E, which have been shown to combat PMS symptoms.[350,351]

Furthermore, raw cacao nibs have a standout mix of magnesium, potassium, iron, vitamin B6, fiber, healthy fats, and protein.[352]

However, it would be best if you didn't reach for conventional chocolate. Most chocolates below 90% cocoa have surprising amounts of refined sugar.

For example, chocolate with 72% cocoa contains 26% sugar[353], which you should avoid if you experi-ence PMS.

Foods to Avoid

Since premenstrual syndrome goes hand in hand with inflammation, it is essential to avoid pro-inflam-matory foods.[354]

And sugar is one of the most pro-inflammatory foods out there. If you suffer from PMS symptoms, avoiding sugar from ovulation to the menstrual phase can make all the difference.

Researchers have found that the fructose in sugar increases the hunger hormone ghrelin, pro-moting cravings.[355]

In addition, research has shown that consumption of sugary drinks is closely related to PMS symptoms.[356]

However, foods and beverages sweetened with sugar and other refined carbohydrates promote inflammation in the body.[357]

Refinement means that foods have been separated from natural fiber, widely processed, and preserved.

Accordingly, here is a summary of these pro-inflammatory foods:

- Bread
- Pasta
- Crackers
- Tortillas
- Cookies
- Cakes
- Pretzels
- Juices
- Sodas (coke etc.)
- Sports drinks
- Energy drinks
- Sweetened tea and coffee beverages

In addition, industrial seed oils are highly inflammatory.[358]

Therefore, for a healthy menstrual cycle, it is vital to avoid the following oils, fried foods, and especially hydrogenated trans fats such as margarine:

- Safflower oil
- Peanut oil
- Corn oil
- Canola oil
- Cottonseed oil
- Soybean oil
- Sunflower oil
- Sesame oil
- Grapeseed oil
- Partially hydrogenated oils

Lastly, alcohol cannot be unmentioned among the worst foods for a healthy period. It distracts the liver from other metabolic or detoxification tasks, such as eliminating excess estrogen, which serves hormonal balance.

Supplements

If you've been reading my blog for a while, you know I'm not a big fan of supplements – they mostly have sugar and various sweeteners mixed in, and the bioavailability is often questionable.

That's why you should prefer natural foods from fatty fish to cruciferous vegetables to nuts during your menstrual cycle.

If you still want to turn to supplements due to severe PMS symptoms, here are the best options on the current market (affiliate links):

- Antarctic Krill Oil (omega-3 fatty acids)
- High Absorption Magnesium (with B6 and E vitamins)
- Women's Premenstrual Support (B6, E, Magnesium, Ginko, Chasteberry)

Your body can absorb the anti-inflammatory omega-3 fatty acids EPA and DHA even better from krill oil than fish oil.[359] And according to studies, regular fish oil already combats period cramps better than ibuprofen.[360]

On top of that, krill oil can help build muscle.

Scientists have shown that magnesium and vitamin B6 are the go-to micronutrients for easing PMS symptoms.[361]

In addition to B6, vitamin E supplementation has also been shown to counteract breast pain, one of the first PMS symptoms.[362]

In the women's premenstrual supplement listed above, the two vitamins are complemented by other vitamins and minerals, which could be beneficial during menstruation.

How to Break a Weight Loss Plateau

Don't despair right away if you've just hit a weight loss plateau for the first time on intermittent fasting.

The causes are as individual as the human body.

To find out how your unique body responds to foods and habits, you need to experiment and listen to it.

If you strictly stick to your intermittent fasting schedule and still have problems shedding excess body fat, you might not be aware of some hidden factors.

However, if you cheat and sugar your tea or drink coffee with milk during your fasting period, don't be surprised if you stall.

You must focus on your diet and scrutinize your lifestyle and routines to achieve your goals.

Here are ten secret hacks to help you break through a plateau on intermittent fasting.

1. Avoid Processed Food

Also, with intermittent fasting, the focus is on fresh, natural food. Those who stick to industrial products from colorful packaging will hardly be successful.

Also, the fitness industry has become a mecca for shelf-stable foods.

Nevertheless, these industrially processed foods contain artificial colors, flavors, preservatives, and other additives that impede healthy metabolic function.[363,364]

Moreover, it doesn't matter if the label says *low-carb, keto, organic,* or *vegan.*

Especially those products aimed at sports or a special diet are mostly highly processed garbage.

Accordingly, added fiber is worthless and cannot dampen blood sugar and insulin spikes like fiber in natural food.

Hence, on intermittent fasting, the consumption of fresh food paves the way to success. So take the time to prepare authentic meals and exchange the protein bar for a free-range egg.

2. Cut Back in Carbs

Even more important than the number of calories consumed is their quality.

With this in mind, carbohydrates, in particular, stimulate insulin production and weight gain most strongly.

However, we should already have eliminated some carbohydrates by crossing processed snacks and other convenience products off the shopping list.

But you don't want to believe that cheap refined carbs are hiding everywhere. For example, you will find them in vinegar, sauces, dressings, mustard, yogurt, etc.

Therefore I can only emphasize again and again that reading labels is mandatory. The food industry is exceptionally creative when it comes to names for sugar.

What ends up on -dextrin, -ose, -syrup, or -extract on the ingredients list is nothing but sugar.

Furthermore, it should be clear that starch is a polysaccharide. Therefore, potatoes, rice, corn, pasta, and bakery goods spike blood sugar and insulin levels.

Farmers use these foods to fatten livestock for a reason. They are a guarantee for weight gain.

Thus, exchanging these carbohydrates for healthy fat makes sense since it hardly raises insulin levels.

3. Focus on Satiety

In contrast to carbohydrate-rich meals, fat-rich meals stimulate the release of satiety hormones much more strongly.

Hormones such as the peptide YY, GLP-1, or leptin send signals to the brain's satiety center – the hypothalamus.[365]

Ghrelin, on the other hand, is a hormone that signals hunger to the hypothalamus. Sugar, especially sweet fructose, stimulates ghrelin release.[366]

That is why it is easy to overeat sweets, while pure fats are challenging for most people.

Accordingly, one study shows that even 5 hours after eating high-fat avocados, people are about 30% less hungry than after other meals.[367]

Natural proteins also contribute significantly to satiety and need plenty of energy to be metabolized. However, humankind hasn't known that proteins stimulate insulin considerably for quite a while.[368]

Therefore, simple low-carb approaches were doomed to fail.

For this reason, you should aim for a medium protein level to lose weight. For intermittent fasting, an energy intake low in carbohydrates, moderate in protein, and rich in healthy fats is ideal.

The bottom line is a ketogenic diet that complements intermittent fasting best, not only because of how our body burns fat.

4. Steer Clear of Lectins

They are often dismissed as harmless, but the scientific burden of proof is overwhelming. Lectins come in countless variations, although you may have only heard of gluten so far.

Plants are not magically resistant to predators. Due to these sticky proteins, they are protected.[369]

Accordingly, lectins can bind to nerve endings in the gut and brain, which can cause inflammation and toxic reactions.[370]

The most crucial factor in weight loss is their ability to bind to insulin and leptin receptors and, thus, cause weight gain.[371]

It is not without reason that lectin-containing foods such as wheat have repeatedly helped humanity build considerable fat reserves for winter.

Since vegetables containing lectin are the focus of industrial agriculture, they can be the well-hidden reason you are not losing weight on intermittent fasting.

As these vegetables are particularly resistant to parasites, they are the preferred varieties for cultivation:

- Cereals and pseudocereals (e.g., quinoa)
- Nightshades (e.g., tomatoes, potatoes, or eggplants)
- Cucurbits (incl. zucchini and cucumbers)
- Legumes (incl. peanuts and cashews)
- Soy

Grains and pseudo-cereals, in particular, should not be on your menu if you want to lose weight.

The greatest evil is whole grain products since particularly aggressive lectins such as wheat germ agglutinin, which endangers intestinal health, are found in the bran.[372]

5. Reduce Stress

Stress is an essential factor people often overlook when weight loss stalls during intermittent fasting.

Nowadays, we are regularly exposed to psychological stressors, and the body releases cortisol more often than is healthy for us.

Cortisol is a steroid hormone crucial for stress reaction – the so-called fight or flight response.

Therefore, cortisol has been evolutionarily essential to prepare the body for fight or flight. For example, to escape the threat of a predator.

After cortisol is released, it increases blood sugar levels. The mobilized energy aims to strengthen the muscles and eventually flee and survive.[373]

The increased blood sugar, in turn, results in an elevated insulin level. Therefore stress directly counteracts the weight loss effect of intermittent fasting.

Besides, it limits metabolic functions such as digestion to focus on surviving.

As permanent stress constantly stimulates insulin secretion, it contributes to weight gain, insulin resistance, and type 2 diabetes.[374]

Furthermore, the fat storage enzyme 11 beta-hydroxysteroid dehydrogenase-1 (HSD) can reactivate inactive cortisol stored in belly fat.

As a result, fat storage within these abdominal cells is stimulated.[375]

6. Get Enough Sleep

Probably the most effective way to counteract stress is to get enough sleep. Conversely, lack of sleep is one of the most significant stressors.

However, about one-third of all working adults now get less than six hours of sleep every night.

In this context, a sleep deprivation and obesity meta-analysis show that less than six hours of sleep increases the risk of weight gain by a whopping 50 percent.[376]

Lack of sleep affects your hormones. For example, it elevates cortisol and ghrelin while lowering leptin levels.

The bottom line is that this sets a vicious circle in motion. While more ghrelin and less leptin trigger increased appetite, cortisol promotes fat storage via insulin.[377]

If you get less than eight hours of sleep daily, you have found a significant reason not to lose weight on intermittent fasting.

7. Do Not Overtrain

Like too little sleep, too much exercise can also stress the body. You can get too much of a good thing, after all.

There is also a healthy limit to working out. People often exceed the healthy limit because exercise is still advertised as the panacea that can magically nullify poor diet choices.

Although exercise is crucial for mental health, diet is the basis for sustainable weight loss.

The most common form of exaggeration is by doing endurance training. And it is precisely this that activates compensatory mechanisms. Those who run a lot will eat a lot.

The exponentially increasing appetite is something I had to witness repeatedly during marathon preparation, in which I always put on weight.

The body reclaims its energy and prepares for more intense energy consumption. Undoubtedly, as biology demands it, you will also overeat if you overdo endurance training.

While healthy training causes acute inflammation, excessive exercise can cause chronic inflammation and stress, counteracting weight loss.[378]

In addition, too much exercise can shift the focus from reproduction to female survival.

Therefore, excessive exercise impairs the release of essential fertility hormones, leading to periods' absence.[379]

Therefore, especially for intermittent fasting beginners, a healthy amount of exercise is purposeful. More than two to three sessions per week are by no means necessary.

8. Stop Drinking Calories

A sports drink after working out and an organic juice for lunch is healthy, isn't it?

Well, not so fast.

Drinks are one of the most common reasons for not losing weight.

No matter how ketogenic your diet is, you'll still lose weight with these liquid meals.

You must avoid sugary drinks such as sodas and juices at all costs.

When you remove the protective dietary fiber from fruits, which are already full of sugar, the blood sugar and insulin will skyrocket.

Juices are not healthy and never will be – no matter how *organic* they are.

You can also overdo it with supposedly healthy things. If you drink every coffee with organic cream or grass-fed butter, this consumed energy will add up throughout the day.

A *Bulletproof Coffee* makes sense if it helps you stay full longer without needing a meal during fasting. After all, you want to burn your body fat instead.

The cornerstones of intermittent fasting are water, tea, and coffee without additives. This way, you prevent calories from entering your body while staying hydrated, which prevents headaches during fasting.

Finally, you must pay attention to the label of all other drinks. Spoiler: Thereby, alleged weight loss drinks often come out as fattening.

By the way, among the worst fatteners are low-fat and protein drinks.

9. Quit Sweeteners

Non-nutritive diet and zero drinks have always enjoyed great popularity. Yet these products cause people to hit a plateau in intermittent fasting repeatedly.

Does zero sugar stand for increased fat burning, as the advertising teaches us? Unfortunately, the reality is different.

Although zero-calorie sweeteners such as aspartame, monk fruit, or stevia do not increase blood glucose levels, they too stimulate insulin secretion.[380,381,382]

For this reason, sweeteners also break the fast.

In addition, they can wipe out gut bacteria that contribute significantly to our health.[383]

Even though sweeteners do not spike blood sugar levels, they make us hungry for more. Diet soda fuels sweet cravings more than drinks with conventional sugar.[384]

It doesn't seem like people who drink diet soda like water are more often overweight – that's a proven fact!

Accordingly, researchers at the University of Texas at San Antonio found that consuming diet soda increases the likelihood of weight gain by 47 percent.[385]

Because of zero-sugar drinks, some people remain unsuccessful even with intermittent fasting. Don't be one of them!

10. Test Ketone Levels

As we know, fasting through ketosis burns fat for energy.

Since there is no food intake during fasting, the body can more easily tap into fat reserves and use the stored energy.

That is why intermittent fasting also aims to achieve the metabolic state of ketosis.

Human bodies react very individually to dietary changes. For this reason, it can help you lose weight to check your ketone levels again and again.

You will get to know your body and its characteristics better.

Accordingly, different foods often hinder ketosis and cause a weight-loss stall for many women.

If you want to precisely know what is good for your intestines, mind, and metabolism, you can also track your meals in a diary.

The more aha-moments you experience, the less often it will be necessary to measure ketone levels.

Finally, the body needs a few weeks to adapt and become fat-adapted.

Therefore, it makes sense to test ketone levels in the blood, especially in the beginning.

In addition, checking them gives you a feeling of certainty about how you react to different foods and what progress you are making.

This way, you can lose weight confidently.

There are four ways to measure ketones in your body (affiliate links):

- Urine test strips
- Blood meter
- Breathalyzer

In ketosis, you can detect the number of ketone bodies in your blood and urine.

With test strips, you measure the ketone bodies in your urine. This method is a quick and the cheapest way to measure ketosis in the short term.

Summarized, you pee on a paper strip that changes color when ketones are detected.

Although ketone test strips are not very accurate, they will give you a general idea of how far you can burn body fat for energy.

When you start intermittent fasting, investing ten dollars in 100 urine test strips is certainly not a mistake to get certainty.

Measuring ketones in the blood, on the other hand, is the most accurate way to measure ketone levels.

As soon as you burn fat efficiently, many ketones travel through the bloodstream, providing energy to cells throughout the body.

The blood test accurately shows how deep you are in ketosis.

You will need a ketone blood meter and appropriate blood test strips to measure ketone levels in your blood.

Since this test method works similarly to how people with diabetes test their blood glucose, you can usually measure your glucose levels at the same time with these devices.

To do this, prick your finger and squeeze a drop of blood onto the test strip, which the meter evaluates.

If the idea of pricking yourself with a needle makes you feel queasy, this method may not be suitable for you.

The newest method for measuring ketone levels is breath testing.

In this, you turn on the ketone meter, let it warm, and then give a breath sample.

A breath meter is more expensive than other ketone tests, but it is a one-time investment. Therefore, you don't have to keep buying more test strips.

It's the only method where you can test indefinitely without incurring additional costs.

However, if you have been drinking alcohol, the ketone levels in your breath will be inaccurate until your body has broken down the alcohol.

Ketone testing has helped many people break through a plateau while practicing intermittent fasting.

That you can explore how your body reacts individually to different foods is a valuable plus.

With this in mind, it should now be clear that combining a ketogenic diet and intermittent fasting 16/8 produces the best weight loss results for many women.

Accordingly, you can also avoid a weight-loss stall by integrating this diet step by step into your eating window.

Boost Fat Burning With Keto

After we already had to emphasize several times how important it is for hormone balance, weight loss, and longevity to focus on healthy fats and reduce carbohydrates during eating periods, here comes the overdue digression.

Rightly so, more and more people are reporting that ketogenic eating brings noticeably better results during intermittent fasting. Why?

Because the keto diet, just like fasting, lowers insulin levels, empties carbohydrate stores, and burns fat through ketosis, making it an ideal match.

In short, the ketogenic diet does nothing but mimic the state of fasting.

The keto diet is a special *low-carb, healthy-fat (LCHF)* diet that forces the body to switch to fat energy sources (ketones).

Since fasting burns your body fat for energy, it's the most ketogenic diet.

To realize the full potential of intermittent fasting through a ketogenic diet, you need a caloric intake of at least 75% fat, 20-25% protein, and 5-10% carbohydrate.

While one gram of fat provides nine calories, one gram of protein or carbohydrates provides four calories, which reduces the absolute amount of fat in proportion.

Accordingly, the meals in grams must consist of only a good 50% of fat. And that can be realized easier than you might think, especially with healthy fats like extra virgin olive oil or grass-fed butter.

Keto builds on the knowledge that even lean proteins can significantly increase insulin levels. This fact was long unknown, dooming classic low-carb diets like the Atkins diet to failure.[386]

Because of decades of public demonizing of fat, low-carb diets were predominantly low-fat. However, fat is the only macronutrient that does not significantly increase insulin production. And that ultimately helps you lose weight.

Because the keto diet does not attempt to do anything other than gain the same benefits as fasting through nutrition, it combines so well with intermittent fasting. By doing so, you can realize the following synergies:

- **Get into ketosis faster:** The ketogenic diet gives you a head start on intermittent fasting, allowing you to tap into body fat for energy sooner and more intensely.

- **Fewer side effects:** The keto diet also reduces possible side effects in the beginning, such as keto flu or upset stomach, that can occur with high-carbohydrate diets during intermittent fasting.

- **More energy:** Because the brain and other organs can use ketones more efficiently than carbohydrates for energy, many people report improved energy, performance, mood, and reduced appetite in the state of ketosis.[387] The increased release of adrenaline during fasting may further support this increase in productivity.[388]

- **Satiety:** After the ketogenic diet helps control appetite and keeps you full longer, you'll find it much easier to adjust to more extended periods without food.

- **Stability:** Due to the so-called fat or keto-adaptation, the body no longer has to constantly switch back and forth between using glucose and fat for energy. This way, you can establish a healthy lifestyle more quickly and permanently while preventing mood swings.

Even if you break your fast with a meal between fasting intervals, you'll still be in ketosis and fasting mode, so to speak, because of the ketogenic diet.

Because of the high-fat-low-carb diet, the body continues as if it were fasting while receiving a tremendously high density of nutrients.

The enhanced fat-burning capabilities of ketosis and the low release of insulin over fasting allow you to achieve and maintain a healthier body weight faster.

It also makes it easier to break a weight-loss stall.

Intermittent fasting likewise trains the body to get used to taking in a day's worth of calories in a shorter time frame, easing digestion and strengthening the intestinal microflora.

When you incorporate intermittent fasting and the ketogenic diet into your daily routine, over time, you learn to eat when you're truly hungry only.

In addition, this combination can sometimes even improve the following health benefits of intermittent fasting:

- Insulin sensitivity
- Fat burning
- Autophagy
- Reduced inflammation
- Memory function
- Gut health

Stall Despite Keto and Fasting

A ketogenic diet gives you an almost unfair advantage. Things get tricky if you can't lose weight despite keto and intermittent fasting.

However, your body is not a weight loss machine that can permanently lose weight. Having that said, stagnation could also have the following reasons:

- **Initial weight loss:** At the beginning of the intermittent fasting, you lost a lot of weight in the form of water retention, and now you wonder why it does not continue at the same pace

- **Approaching target weight:** If you have already lost significant weight, weight loss will slow down. The closer you reach your target weight, you often experience a standstill.

- **Thyroid problems:** If you have reached this point, you may experience thyroid or adrenal gland issues and immediately contact your doctor.

Sample Meal Plan

When you start intermittent fasting, you will surely think about how it will affect your body, metabolism, and mind.

When it comes to intermittent fasting, the daily plan that has proven to be the easiest for most women to integrate into their daily routine is the 16/8 method.

In addition, its simple rules allow beginners to get off to the best possible start.

Since experience has shown it to be the easiest and most effective, my sample plan omits breakfast. Moreover, most people like to eat dinner with their family.

In any case, it makes sense to get 8 hours of sleep during the fasting period. This way, you shorten the fast to only 8 hours a day, which is only half.

For this reason, I do not recommend skipping lunch. Nevertheless, some people have successfully done this because of their unusual daily schedules.

The following 16/8 meal plan is deliberately low in carbohydrates, making it a guarantor of exceptional fat burning.

Moreover, these are dishes that you can easily prepare since they usually require only three ingredients and no preparation:

Monday

- **Breakfast:** Fasting
- **Lunch:** Avocado tuna salad with egg
- **Dinner:** Pork chops baked with cheese and steamed broccoli in olive oil

Tuesday

- **Breakfast:** Fasting
- **Lunch:** Chicken mayonnaise salad with cucumber, avocado, onion, and walnuts
- **Dinner:** Roasted chicken legs with mashed cauliflower

Wednesday

- **Breakfast:** Fasting
- **Lunch:** Ground beef lettuce wraps with cheddar cheese, onion, and bell pepper
- **Dinner:** Chicken stuffed with cream cheese, served with roasted asparagus

Thursday

- **Breakfast:** Fasting
- **Lunch:** Roasted pork belly, served with steamed kohlrabi
- **Dinner:** Mackerel fried in coconut oil with kale and toasted pine nuts

Friday

- **Breakfast:** Fasting
- **Lunch:** Grilled salmon with a salad of leafy greens, feta, and tomato
- **Dinner:** Ribeye steak, butter, and coleslaw

Saturday

- **Breakfast:** Fasting
- **Lunch:** Chicken salad with olive oil, feta cheese, olives, and lettuce
- **Dinner:** Pasture-raised beef burger (no bun) with tomato, onion, cheese, and kale

Sunday

- **Breakfast:** Fasting
- **Lunch:** Garlic butter steak with mushrooms and asparagus
- **Dinner:** Cheese bowl tacos with guacamole

This weekly plan deliberately does not include snacks, as not having snacks in between meals helps you lose weight by lowering insulin levels.

However, snacks are not forbidden during the 8-hour eating period, as long as you don't overdo it. You can find the best snacks to buy and make yourself on www.mentalfoodchain.com\keto-snacks-recipes\.

Weekly Schedule Overview

This subchapter illustrates all the essential methods we analyzed in PART II.

This way, you get the necessary overview of how the eating and fasting windows of the different plans are distributed throughout the day and week.

These page-sized diagrams should serve you as a visual basis for how you can put time-restricted eating into practice step by step.

We start with 12/12 intermittent fasting since it's the most straightforward method with the slightest need to change a daily schedule without Intermittent Fasting.

After that comes the crescendo method, which will help you gently transition to the 16/8 schedule.

The weekly plan with a standardized eating window of 8 hours should finally manifest the lifestyle that you can implement in the long run to optimize your health sustainably.

Intermittent Fasting 12/12

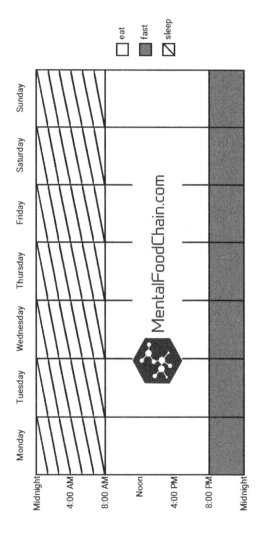

Crescendo Fasting

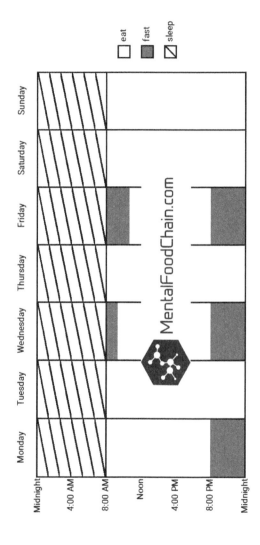

Intermittent Fasting 16/8

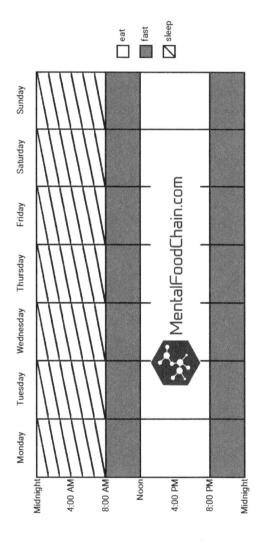

30-Day Intermittent Fasting Challenge

Changing diets can feel like a monumental task.

Changes associated with it usually seem intimidating at first.

Plus, it can feel overwhelming as you think about when, how often, and what to eat, or what exercise can help with weight loss and to what extent.

In addition, a new diet always comes with a certain feeling of insecurity.

And it is precisely this unpleasant feeling that I want to take away from you with this fasting challenge.

The 30-day plan combines all the essential new factors you have already learned about in this book.

So you can start intermittent fasting confidently, without risking your health or fretting about annoying mistakes.

In short, I've invested time and experience into this fasting challenge so you can take all the guesswork out of losing weight.

On top of that, it takes the tricky decisions away from you, ensuring that you don't lose motivation as you start your 16/8 intermittent fasting plan.

After mastering this challenge, you will be convinced that the 16/8 schedule is the easiest way for women to lose weight effectively without starving themselves.

For this 30-day plan, you don't have to prepare 90 exotic recipes, portion them, calculate the calories you consume, or follow other complicated rules.

After that, you'll realize that intermittent fasting is not witchcraft but a lifestyle most people can easily integrate into their daily work routine.

The best part is that the challenge is free and can be done by almost anyone at any time.

If you want to improve your health, the following small daily challenges are just the thing to get you started today.

I've made the daily activities as simple as possible so that you can make small changes, step by step, to get you closer to your wellness weight.

On the one hand, this 30-day plan will get you used to intermittent fasting gradually and effortlessly. And on the other hand, it will help you become aware of habits that may have unconsciously prevented you from losing weight.

Accordingly, the challenge will slowly introduce you to the 16/8 method via 12/12 and crescendo fasting. This approach to intermittent fasting exactly is what we were able to derive as ideal in the book's second part.

This way, you can start intermittent fasting without fear of messing up your cycle.

Each week of the Challenge has a specific theme that will get you closer to your goals:

1. Drink Awareness

2. Food Awareness

3. Mindfulness

4. Fat Burning

Each small challenge will help you improve your relationship with food, regulate your appetite naturally, and establish activities that relieve stress without overwhelming you.

Monthly Schedule

	Sunday	Monday	Tuesday	Wednesday	Thursday	Friday	Saturday
Drink Awareness	**1** Eat: 12 AM - 8 PM / No snacking after 8 PM	**2** Eat: 8 AM - 8 PM / No more juices, smoothies, diet sodas, etc	**3** Eat: 8 AM - 8 PM / Drink a full glass of water every day after getting up	**4** Eat: 10 AM - 8 PM / Exclusively water/coffee/tea before 10 AM	**5** Eat: 8 AM - 8 PM / Swap Breakfast for Bulletproof Coffee/Tea	**6** Eat: Noon - 8 PM / No more milk/sugar/sweeteners in coffee/tea	**7** Eat: 8 AM - 8 PM / Enjoy the weekend, but do not reward with junk food
Food Awareness	**8** Eat: 8 AM - 8 PM / Reflect the previous week	**9** Eat: 10 AM - 8 PM / Start reading labels and pay attention to sugars/oils	**10** Eat: 8 AM - 8 PM / Buy raw and avoid processed foods	**11** Eat: Noon - 8 PM / Swap classic side dishes for green vegetables	**12** Eat: 8 AM - 8 PM / Limit snacks (nuts/berries) to noon - 8 PM	**13** Eat: Noon - 8 PM / Test ketones with test strips or a meter	**14** Eat: 8 AM - 8 PM / Enjoy the weekend, but do not reward with junk food
Mindfulness	**15** Eat: 8 AM - 8 PM / Reflect the previous week	**16** Eat: Noon - 8 PM / Introduce a walk after dinner	**17** Eat: Noon - 8 PM / Avoid social media while fasting	**18** Eat: Noon - 8 PM / Implement a 10 min morning routine Yoga/Mediation	**19** Eat: Noon - 8 PM / Turn off the Wi-Fi and dim the lights every day at 10 PM	**20** Eat: Noon - 8 PM / Test ketones with test strips or a meter	**21** Eat: Noon - 8 PM / Enjoy the weekend, but do not reward with junk food
Fat Burning	**22** Eat: Noon - 8 PM / Reflect the previous week	**23** Eat: Noon - 8 PM / Start the day with a fasted workout (~10 min.)	**24** Eat: Noon - 8 PM / Cook with healthy fats (ghee/virgin coconut/olive oil)	**25** Eat: Noon - 8 PM / Take a run in a fasted state before dinner	**26** Eat: Noon - 8 PM / Eat ketogenic throughout the day	**27** Eat: 2 PM - 8 PM / Test ketones with test strips or a meter	**28** Eat: Noon - 8 PM / Enjoy the weekend, but do not reward with junk food
	29 Eat: Noon - 8 PM / Reflect previous week	**30** Eat: 5 PM - 8 PM / Test final ketone levels					

1. Drink Awareness Week

Although people are constantly racking their brains over food, most serious mistakes happen while drinking. Countless beverages can deprive you of any chance of reaching your target weight. Put an end to that now!

Day 1

The first day is simple. You are going to stop eating at 8:00 PM. Not snacking is the first significant milestone in introducing you to a successful intermittent fasting routine.

Today, try to avoid snacks in between meals. Therefore, you will start only drinking tap water, mineral water, coffee, or tea from now on.

Ask yourself if you are actually hungry. Maybe you're just stressed, worried, or bored. It might also help if you grab your shoes and go for a walk instead of grabbing a snack.

Check and record your waist circumference, body weight, and BMI today. This way, you can analyze the results at the end of the challenge.

Day 2

Today we are going to eliminate the secret killers of all weight loss ambitions:

- Juices of all kinds, no matter how organic
- Regular, diet, and zero sodas
- Smoothies (sugar without fiber)
- Sports drinks (sweeteners and sugars)
- Low fat and fasting drinks (insulin)
- Energy drinks (absolute garbage)

Your body will thank you!

Day 3

After getting up, a glass (250 ml) of water will help you start intermittent fasting and is also obligatory for a healthy fluid balance.

It is crucial to drink the water before any coffee.

Day 4

Today is the first day of crescendo fasting to shorten the eating window.

To summarize, today you are not supposed to eat a meal as soon as you get up, just because most other people do the same.

For this reason, only unsweetened tea or coffee and water is allowed before 10 AM.

Day 5

Today we take a significant step toward the 16/8 schedule.

Instead of breakfast, you will have a high-fat drink that can fill you up without significantly increasing insulin levels.

This fat fasting extends the time in which you can burn fat efficiently.

We use a Bulletproof Coffee or Tea (same recipe with tea instead of coffee).

The keto-friendly butter coffee is also famous for intermittent fasting.

The essential aspect of any Bulletproof Coffee is the addition of healthy fats. Therefore, a Bulletproof Coffee is different from an ordinary coffee with milk.

The classic recipe for Bulletproof Coffee, which you will find at the end of this challenge, includes black coffee and two essential ingredients:

- MCT oil or virgin coconut oil
- Pastured butter or ghee

While these pure fats do not stop ketosis, they do impair autophagy.

For this reason, Bulletproof Coffee is just a jumpstart to help you get used to longer fasting windows more easily in the beginning.

Throughout this fasting challenge, you will unlearn morning hunger anyway. Then starting aids will become obsolete.

Day 6

The end of the week eliminates more hidden bad guys that can prevent you from losing weight.

Yes, even non-nutritive sweeteners fuel cravings, stimulate insulin production, and prevent you from losing weight.[389,390,391,392,393,394]

Therefore, from this day of the intermittent fasting challenge, the following additives in coffee, tea, or other beverages are taboo:

- Milk
- Sugar
- Sweeteners

In addition, this day is the first of the challenge in which you should follow the classic 16/8 pattern.

Day 7

On the weekend, you can eat relaxedly utilizing a 12/12 schedule.

However, that doesn't mean you should stuff yourself with donuts, burgers, and fries for two days.

Take a little mindfulness into the weekend and avoid unnecessary sweetened and low-fat diet drinks.

2. Food Awareness Week

No matter what approach you take to improve your health or shed five pounds to fit back into your old pants, you can't avoid one cornerstone: Natural foods rich in micronutrients.

When you fast clean, you not only save yourself from bloating, inflammation, cravings, and blemished skin but also lose weight sustainably without the yo-yo effect.

That's why the second week of the challenge aims to raise awareness of the additives the food industry smuggles into our food to make it cheaper to produce and shelf-stable.

Day 8

After your first fasting experience, take a few minutes to reflect on old eating habits and set goals for the week.

What might have been holding you back from losing weight so far? How can you overcome this hurdle in the future?

Write down your thoughts, try to live more in the present, and appreciate the novelties and insights of each day accordingly.

Day 9

A work week couldn't start any better with a focus on eating more consciously.

When you start reading labels, you won't be able to escape the amazement of what's hiding in some foods.

The food industry mixes in sugar wherever possible because it is eight times as addictive as cocaine.[395]

Furthermore, *big food* is creative in inventing names for sugar to prevent it from being the first ingredient on the package.

Anything that ends in -dextrin, -ose, -syrup, or -extract among the ingredients is most likely sugar.

Sucrose, conventional table sugar, is not a simple sugar. In addition to glucose, it contains a much sweeter sugar molecule called fructose.

And we know that fructose inhibits the satiety hormone leptin and stimulates the hunger hormone ghrelin.[396]

Eating sugary foods during your last meal can make it harder for you to fast the next day. Highly processed foods do not make you feel full but make you hungry faster.

Like sugar, refined seed oils have now made it into colorful packaging.

They act as cheap flavor carrier alternatives to natural fats.

The trend of swapping natural saturated fats for industrial omega-6 fats is fattening and promotes inflammation, cardiovascular disease, and mortality in general.[397]

Using these harmful oils for frying is also the main argument against eating out.

Take extra virgin olive or coconut oil with your last meal today instead of sugar to get satiated.

This day has a 10-hour eating window as part of the crescendo method.

Day 10

In addition to the arguments above, artificial colors and flavors,[398] preservatives, and other chemical additives[399] are a reason to buy real food.

Natural, whole foods not made up of multiple ingredients should be the cornerstone of any rudimentary healthy diet.

Although this basic rule is self-explanatory, many people today lack the necessary awareness.

Day 10 of the challenge allows you to eat for 12 hours from morning to night.

Day 11

Try to eat only lunch and dinner on this day.

The conventional pairing of fatty acids and polysaccharides like starches on your plate works against weight loss.

While fat brings more energy into the body, glucose ensures that energy is stored efficiently through insulin release.

In contrast to classic side dishes such as potatoes, pasta, or bread, a fundamentally different type of carbohydrate predominates in green vegetables: Dietary fiber.

While simple and multiple sugars raise blood sugar and insulin levels, fiber reduces their rise.[400]

Your first options in today's side dishes, therefore, are:

- Brussels sprouts
- Broccoli
- Cauliflower
- Asparagus
- Cabbage

Feel free to add grass-fed butter or extra virgin olive oil to the vegetables to help with satiety.

Day 12

In moderation, the right snacks can also be healthy. While today is the last time you may eat throughout the day, try limiting snacks to the afternoon.

Allowed are various nuts as healthy sources of fat (peanuts and cashews are neither nuts nor healthy fats!) and those fruits that contain the least sugar: Berries and citrus fruits.

Day 13

Now that you're fasting at 16/8 again, it's time to see how well your body has adapted to burning fat for energy.

Intermittent fasting also aims to achieve a state of ketosis, where the body uses fat instead of glucose for fuel.

Although experienced fasting enthusiasts may feel as if they are in ketosis by paying attention to their body's reactions, we want to check your progress more closely.

You can determine ketone levels through test strips, a blood meter, or a breathalyzer (affiliate links).

While urine tests are cheaper, blood tests provide the most accurate results.

If no ketones show up in your test results today, don't despair.

It may well take the full 30 days for you to become fat-adapted. In the case of solid insulin resistance, it can also take considerably longer.

Accordingly, it is already a success if you can detect increased ketone levels during the challenge.

Therefore, we will now perform this measurement every Friday before lunch and before breaking the last fast to measure the first possible success.

After Friday is the start of the weekend, there are no additional tasks. Enjoy the weekend!

Day 14

On the weekend, you eat again relaxed utilizing a 12/12 interval.

Take your new food awareness into the weekend and avoid unnecessary, highly processed foods.

3. Mindfulness Week

Since awareness is the sub-theme of this fasting challenge, the development of mindfulness cannot be missing.

Mindfulness means nothing more than living the present moment judgment-free and consciously. In short, we want to perceive the now in a more focused way and let distractions pass us by so that we don't mentally digress.

Mindfulness-based practices have one primary purpose, to reduce stress and thus cortisol levels.

Stress inevitably arises at work, during everyday interactions, and during leisure time.

It is the biggest silent killer of all weight loss ambitions. You can integrate mindfulness into your daily routine with surprisingly simple habits, increase your well-being, and lose weight more efficiently.

Day 15

On Sunday, take a few minutes to reflect on your key learnings from the previous week.

Write down three aha-moments that you think could fundamentally change your relationship with food for the better.

Day 16

In the second half of this fasting challenge, we finally move to the 16/8 schedule. You have completed the introductory phase, and from now on, you'll eat every day only from noon until 8:00 PM.

Today's task is simple but effective. Maybe you have already practiced it a time or two during a COVID lockdown.

Walking after dinner will help you relax and significantly lowers blood glucose levels.

If you have a blood meter, you can compare the readings before and after the walk and witness your effectiveness.

Day 17

Avoid consuming social media from 9:00 AM until noon.

Charming images of food abound on social media, making it much more challenging to persevere while fasting.

Focus on work and marvel at how productive mornings can be without breakfast and social media.

Day 18

Meditation and yoga are the main pillars of *Mindfulness-Based Stress Reduction Techniques (MBSR)*.

The main idea behind mindfulness-based stress reduction is to live fully in the present moment through repetitive awareness exercises.

It is a lifestyle change aimed at escaping the millwheels of time.

Mindfulness-based practices can reduce stress symptoms while increasing sleep and quality of life.[401]

According to research, highly stressed individuals may benefit from meditation to reduce stress.[402]

Yoga, in turn, can reduce cortisol levels, blood pressure, resting heart rate, heart rate variability, and blood sugar.[403]

Choose one of the two methods as your morning routine, which you will maintain throughout the rest of the challenge.

For the first option, I recommend an app that allows you to get started immediately through guided meditations without prior knowledge.

YouTube gives you almost limitless options for 10-minute yoga sessions in the morning. With most of the videos for beginners, you can get started immediately without any prior knowledge.

Day 19

Screens are signaling daytime to our bodies due to their blue light.

That's why the hunger hormone ghrelin and stress hormone cortisol rise again after 10 PM, making it difficult for us to sleep for the next few hours.

This fact even goes so far that researchers have found a correlation between the duration and intensity of light and BMI or body weight.[404]

Fortunately, mobile devices' new night light modes can filter blue light and reduce the stimulating effect.

For PCs, I recommend a software application that adjusts the screen's blue light radiation to match the rhythm of daylight.

But that's only half the story. As long as you're mentally active and in work mode, you'll tend to delay sleep.

The best trick is to use a timer for your Wi-Fi router and set it for 10 PM.

Although it will take some effort to implement this, it will give you a new day with renewed energy, giving you better results in your tasks.

Day 20

Measure the ketone level through test strips, a blood meter, or a breathalyzer before breaking the fast at noon.

How did you progress compared to the previous week?

If so, do you already feel more energized in general?

Day 21

Starting today, you will eat exclusively in the 8 hours of the classic 16/8 method, even on weekends.

Try to do your 10-minute mindfulness-based routine on weekends until the end of the Challenge.

4. Fat Burning Week

The last week of the 30-day intermittent fasting challenge is about getting the most out of the final sprint.

That means we'll finish by incorporating activities that aren't mandatory for intermittent fasting but can help you optimize health and weight loss.

In short, you'll get a taste of the ketogenic diet and exercise this week.

If you read my blog, you know that intermittent fasting doesn't require you to spend your spare time at the gym. Instead, minimal but wise exercise can significantly improve your results and well-being.

However, the ketogenic diet will give you a guaranteed jump-start regarding fat burning and weight loss.

Day 22

Again, take time this Sunday to reflect.

How did you like the activity after dinner? Do you get tired and relaxed sooner when you dim the lights and avoid the blue light of screens in the evening?

Reflect on whether mindfulness-based habits make you more serene during your daily work routine.

Day 23

This week is designed to show you how to properly combine intermittent fasting and exercise to burn maximum fat with minimal effort.

According to an analysis of randomized studies, exercise in a fasted state increases the breakdown of fatty tissue while stimulating peripheral fat burning. The result is increased fat utilization and weight loss.[405]

Start your day with a little workout to help you get the fat-burning going. For the classic 8-minute abs workout on Youtube, you don't need any equipment, and you don't even need 10 minutes.

The 8 minutes can be easily found, for example, by refraining from looking at your smartphone in the morning.

Day 24

Unlike carbohydrates, pure fats trigger almost no blood sugar or insulin response. Moreover, they make you feel fuller for longer.

Cook and refine your meals today with healthy fats such as virgin coconut, olive and avocado oil, grass-fed butter, and ghee.

Also, include fatty fish such as salmon or mackerel, olives, avocados, pecans, macadamias, brazil nuts, or walnuts in your meals.

Day 25

Exercising while fasted offers health benefits.

This way, you can burn fat faster as well as activate autophagy.

Therefore, go for a run after work before eating anything, even if it's just a snack.

We want to aim for a run of about 45 minutes. Try to last at least 30 minutes.

The pace is not important at all. Running slower tends to be better for getting in shape sustainably.

If you can't go any longer, try walking at a brisk pace for at least the planned duration.

Day 26

Even though following a specific diet is not mandatory to lose weight with intermittent fasting, it has been shown that it allows for better results due to blood sugar regulation.

In my diet plan above, you will find countless recipe ideas, as all the dishes in it are suitable for a ketogenic diet.

Pick a day or switch entirely to the diet plan if you feel comfortable.

Day 27

Towards the end of the challenge, we want to reduce your daily eating window a bit if you feel up to it.

Try an 18- to 20-hour overnight fast. Always pay attention to how you feel, and stop if you get dizzy.

Friday is suitable for this experiment, as ideally, you will work through it longer without a lunch break and go home earlier.

Measure the ketone level by test strips, a blood meter, or a breathalyzer before eating.

Is there already progress compared to the previous week?

Were you more productive at work than usual by closing time today?

Day 28

On our last Saturday of the challenge, it would help if you avoided unnecessary junk food and not forgot about the mindfulness routine and the 16/8 rhythm.

Day 29

What did you like and not like about the past week?

Were the healthy fats able to regulate your appetite and stop cravings?

Do you see added value in accommodating a 10-minute exercise session two to three days a week? Has the combination of a ketogenic diet and exercise given you the drive you may have been lacking in your daily life?

Treat yourself to a hearty dinner of fatty fish and lots of olive oil today before your last long-distance fast tomorrow.

Day 30

Today is the final spurt. Skip lunch on the last day!

Drink enough tap water, mineral water, unsweetened black coffee, or green tea. This way, you will keep hunger at bay.

Before dinner, measure the effect of 21 hours without food on your blood ketone levels.

Afterward, congratulate yourself. You have completed the 30-Day Intermittent Fasting Challenge!

What changes did you notice in your body? How has your relationship with food changed? Do you feel healthier and more vibrant than before? Do your clothes fit better? Have you lost body weight, waist circumference, or BMI?

Write down your results, reflect on what key insights you want to take into your everyday life, and tell friends about them.

Recipe: Bulletproof Coffee

Bulletproof Coffee, *Butter Coffee,* or *Keto Coffee*, is an energizing drink made from high-quality fats and coffee beans.

Bulletproof Coffee can sharpen your mental focus when you initially struggle to concentrate while fasting.

Since it's full of healthy fats, it can also replace a meal now and then when time is in short supply.

Due to its performance-enhancing effects, Bulletproof Coffee has become a staple in intermittent fasting and ketogenic diets and among athletes and other ambitious people.

MCTs are responsible for much of Butter Coffee's effect.

MCT stands for medium-chain triglycerides. These are medium-chain fatty acids that occur mainly in coconut oil.

Therefore, although high-quality MCT oil (affiliate link) is derived from coconut oil, it contains a significantly higher MCT concentration.

Because of their shorter chain length, MCTs are metabolized and used by the body more rapidly than other fats.[406]

They are more readily converted to ketones than other fats, supporting intermittent fasting.[407]

Together with the caffeine in coffee, they boost metabolism and fat burning.[408,409]

In addition, grass-fed butter and MCTs help people stay full longer,[410] as they stimulate the release of satiety hormones, which have been shown to reduce food intake.[411]

The first Bulletproof Coffee was created by biohacker *Dave Asprey*. In recent years, however, a variety of versions of the high-fat, sugar-free coffee have evolved, such as the following recipe:

- **2½ tbsp coffee** freshly ground

- **1-2 tbsp MCT oil** or coconut oil

- **1-2 T tbsp grass-fed ghee** or butter

Brew a cup of coffee using 2 ½ tablespoons of freshly ground coffee beans.

Add one teaspoon to 2 tablespoons of MCT oil. Start with one teaspoon and work up to 1-2 tablespoons over several days.

Add 1-2 tablespoons of grass-fed butter or ghee (affiliate link).

Mix everything in a blender for 20-30 seconds until it looks like a creamy latte.

Makes one cup

Frequently Asked Questions

1. What are time windows for intermittent fasting?

Intermittent fasting has many methods and schedules. The times for time-restricted eating are usually given in the fasting period/eating period, such as 16/8.

2. What are the methods of intermittent fasting?

In intermittent fasting, there is the 16/8, 14/10, 23/1, or crescendo method. There are also the 6:1 and 5:2 diets. You can find the details in another book of this series: Intermittent Fasting 101 (affiliate link).

3. Is milk allowed during intermittent fasting?

Since milk contains lactose and milk proteins, it is not allowed during intermittent fasting. These nutrients increase blood sugar and insulin levels and break the fast.

4. What foods are allowed during intermittent fasting?

No food is eaten during the fasting period. However, coffee and tea without milk and sugar are allowed.

For beginners, exceptions such as Bulletproof Coffee or broth have proven effective for getting used to more extended fasting periods.

5. What should I eat during intermittent fasting?

A tremendous success in intermittent fasting is achieved with a low-carb diet such as the ketogenic diet, promoting fat burning.

6. What breaks an intermittent fast?

Meals, sweeteners, soda, soft drinks, juices, coffee with milk, or menthol cigarettes interrupt intermittent fasting.

7. Can I smoke while fasting?

During intermittent fasting, you can smoke self-rolled cigarettes with natural tobacco. During prolonged therapeutic fasting, you should not smoke because it counteracts the ambition of detoxification.

8. What mistakes can be made during intermittent fasting?

Common mistakes in intermittent fasting are milk and sugar in coffee, too little salt, no exercise, or a high carbohydrate diet.

9. Why am I not losing weight with intermittent fasting 16/8?

Many people do not lose weight during intermittent fasting because they eat processed foods, lots of carbohydrates or too little fat, drink juices and diet soda, or sleep too little.

10. How does intermittent fasting work in the body?

According to studies, intermittent fasting improves memory, life expectancy, immune function, muscle gain, metabolism, and mood.

11. Is intermittent fasting good for metabolism?

Intermittent fasting boosts metabolism and fat burning, according to numerous studies.

12. How long does it take for intermittent fasting to work?

It can take 3-6 weeks for the body to relearn how to burn fat efficiently through intermittent fasting.

13. Can intermittent fasting be dangerous?

Intermittent fasting cannot be dangerous for perfectly healthy people. Nevertheless, you should always consult your trusted physician before changing your diet.

14. How long do I have to fast to activate autophagy?

According to studies, autophagy starts after about 14 hours. Exercise, a ketogenic diet, and certain foods can speed up the process.

15. How much weight do I lose with intermittent fasting?

It depends on how much excess weight you carry around. Correctly done, you can reach any realistic target weight with intermittent fasting.

16. How fast can I lose weight with intermittent fasting?

You will notice the first significant weight loss within a week when water depots in the body are emptied. For efficient fat burning, your body may need 3-6 weeks.

17. How effective is the 16/8 diet?

Because this method forces the body to empty carbohydrate stores and tap into body fat for energy, the 16/8 diet can be very effective. The fewer carbohydrates you eat during the eating periods, the more effective.

18. How many calories should I eat during 16/8 intermittent fasting?

Intermittent fasting sets the hormonal course for weight loss. Accordingly, it is not a conventional diet based on calorie counting and portion control. The average daily requirement is enough to lose weight with it.

19. How do I start with intermittent fasting?

You start intermittent fasting by stopping to eat breakfast and snacks. Moreover, when drinking, you limit yourself to water, tea, and coffee without sweeteners or other additives.

20. How many meals should I eat during intermittent fasting?

The classic 16/8 daily plan includes two big meals: lunch and dinner.

21. Which type of intermittent fasting is the best?

The 16/8 method has proven to be the best method for most people, as it is straightforward to integrate into everyday life.

22. what happens in the body after 12 hours of fasting?

After 12 hours of fasting, insulin levels drop, and carbohydrate stores in the body can be depleted.

23. What happens in the body after 14 hours of fasting?

According to studies, 14 hours of fasting is when autophagy starts to kick in.

24. What to eat after 16 hours of fasting?

After fasting, bone broth, fish, chicken, avocados, or cooked cruciferous vegetables are excellent foods.

25. is fruit allowed during intermittent fasting?

As a general rule, no food is eaten during the fasting window. Fruit is not helpful during intermittent fasting because of the high amounts of glucose and fructose. Small amounts of berries are acceptable during the eating period.

26. Why not use dietary supplements during intermittent fasting?

Food supplements are highly processed, often contain sweeteners, and hinder weight loss. Also, it should be the highest premise to take nutrients from natural food when practicing intermittent fasting.

27. Can I combine intermittent fasting and bodybuilding?

For decades, bodybuilders have been using classic 16/8 intermittent fasting to reduce fat while gaining lean mass.

28. Does intermittent fasting make me lose muscle?

Contrary to popular belief, intermittent fasting dramatically increases the release of growth hormone that protects lean mass during fasting and helps build muscle.

29. Does intermittent fasting work without exercise?

Of course, intermittent fasting can work without exercise. However, working out helps empty carbohydrate stores and thus get into fat burning faster.

30. Can intermittent fasting be combined with HIIT training?

Healthy people can combine intermittent fasting with high-intensity interval training (HIIT). According to recent studies, HIIT is particularly good at enhancing the health benefits of intermittent fasting.

31. When to exercise during intermittent fasting?

To promote muscle growth through intermittent fasting, you must train during the fasting period and eat only afterward.

32. What happens in the body when you do not eat for 16 hours?

If you regularly do not eat for 16 hours, the body can use stored fat for energy and renew broken cell parts.

33. What is the benefit of 16/8 intermittent fasting?

Intermittent fasting offers time, money, flexibility, fat burning, improved metabolism, and reduces inflammation and diseases in general.

34. How much can I lose in a week with Intermittent Fasting?

In the first week, you can lose about 3 kg with intermittent fasting after emptying the carbohydrate stores that bind large amounts of water in the body.

35. How does the body react to intermittent fasting?

Besides allowing the body to burn more fat gradually, intermittent fasting lowers insulin levels, which reduces the risk of diabetes and cardiovascular disease.

36. How long should you do intermittent fasting?

How long you fast intermittently is entirely up to you. 16/8 intermittent fasting is very popular because it only requires skipping breakfast and snacks. You can also fast for a whole day during the week and not on other days.

37. Is intermittent fasting good for the gut?

Intermittent fasting has been shown to improve intestinal health. Accordingly, it reduces harmful gut bacteria and inflammation.

38. Can you combine Intermittent Fasting with Low-Carb?

You can combine intermittent fasting with low-carb and achieve even better results because both approaches are based on lowering insulin and thus burning body fat.

39. How do you know you are in ketosis?

A safe and straightforward option is urine test strips for about as little as ten bucks per 100-piece pack.

40. When do you lose weight with intermittent fasting?

With intermittent fasting, you lose weight during the fasting period (usually overnight) because it requires your body to tap into fat deposits as a primary energy source.

41. Which hormones prevent weight loss?

Elevated levels of insulin, cortisol, ghrelin, and neuropeptide Y can prevent weight loss.

42. Which hormones influence weight?

Storage, satiety, stress, and sex hormones can affect weight. The most critical hormones in weight loss are insulin, leptin, and cortisol.

43. Which hormone is a fat killer?

Glucagon and leptin are the hormones most likely to be fat killers. While glucagon stimulates fat loss, leptin signals your body not to build extra fat reserves.

44. Which hormones produce belly fat?

In addition to the primary fat-storage hormone insulin, the stress hormone cortisol leads to increased belly fat.

45. Why do I still feel hungry after eating?

Because carbohydrates, especially sugar, reduce the satiety hormone leptin and increase the hunger hormone ghrelin, you still feel hungry after eating.

46. How can you lower ghrelin?

With a low-carbohydrate, high-fat diet, you can lower ghrelin and increase the release of satiety hormones.

47. how can I lose weight with leptin?

Leptin helps you lose weight because this hormone regulates body fat: If you have eaten enough, your body sends leptin to your brain to tell you that there is enough energy and you are full.

48. Can fasting affect the menstrual cycle?

More extended periods of fasting can affect the menstrual cycle due to severe calorie reduction, which is why shorter fasting windows, such as the 16/8 method, have proven effective for women.

49. Can intermittent fasting affect the period?

Intermittent fasting methods with shorter fasting windows, such as crescendo fasting or 16/8, are unlikely to affect the period. However, fasting for several days can affect a woman's cycle because of the extreme calorie restriction.

50. Can therapeutic fasting influence the period?

Since therapeutic fasting, unlike intermittent fasting, lasts for several days, it can affect periods due to this long-term calorie reduction.

51. Is it possible to eat during the period without gaining weight?

You can eat during your period without gaining weight by avoiding refined carbohydrates like baked goods and eating natural fats and proteins like fish.

52. Can a diet cause missed periods?

You may miss your period if a diet results in a severe calorie deficit.

53. Is intermittent fasting stressful for the body?

Intermittent fasting, like exercise, is healthy stress for the body, provided it is done at the right level.

54. What causes estrogen dominance?

The most common causes of estrogen dominance are sugar, a high-carbohydrate diet, body fat, plastic packaging, skin creams, and chronic stress.

55. When is estrogen dominance present?

Estrogen dominance is when there is either too much estrogen or too little progesterone in the body.

56. What are the symptoms of estrogen dominance?

Symptoms of estrogen dominance range from mild mood swings to weight gain to abnormal uterine bleeding.

57. What can you do for estrogen dominance?

You can combat estrogen dominance naturally by avoiding carbohydrates, stress, plastic packaging, and skin creams.

58. When is PMS worst?

Although the onset of PMS can be very individual, the worst symptoms are usually experienced toward the end of the luteal phase (day 15-28 of the menstrual cycle) before menstruation.

59. What can you do about PMS?

Reducing stress, carbohydrates, sugar, and eating foods with omega-3 fatty acids, magnesium, and vitamins B6 and E can relieve PMS symptoms.

60. How many PMS symptoms are there?

There are 40 PMS symptoms, of which the most common are cramps, breast pain, depression, anxiety, fatigue, cravings, and sleep problems.

61. What percentage of women have PMS?

Researchers estimate that 80-90% experience a symptom at least once, and 47.8% of women worldwide suffer from PMS.

Conclusion

In summary, hormones are the key to sustainable health. Fortunately, they are elementary lifestyle factors that can bring them into balance.

Intermittent fasting 16/8 is the intervention that brings the most outstanding results for hormone balance with the least effort.

Moreover, this method's popularity is because it can be integrated almost effortlessly into any daily routine.

An optimal balance of eating and fasting is why this method guarantees success for most women.

It regulates the hormone balance with minor changes so that the metabolism becomes healthier step by step and enables efficient fat burning.[412]

Since 16/8 fasting is not an extreme method with restrictive rules, it does not upset fertility hormones.

Instead, general factors such as excessive exercise, stress, and caloric restriction can disrupt the menstrual cycle. These are not specifics of intermittent fasting.

It is widespread for women to combine intermittent fasting with severe calorie restriction and a tremendous amount of exercise when they begin.

Stress caused by this can affect the cycle of the female body.

For this reason, intermittent fasting methods have been developed for women that provide a gentle start, such as crescendo fasting.

If you want to start intermittent fasting worry-free, this book's 30-Day Challenge is the place to start.

It takes you by the hand and guides you step by step into a lifestyle you can maintain without struggling.

What's more, you don't have to deny much. Intermittent fasting is not a conventional diet where you have to count calories.

Moreover, you don't risk your reproductive health by simply postponing your food intake.[413]

In addition, it eliminates annoying yo-yo dieting.[414]

However, it would help if you remembered that intermittent fasting is mainly about meal timing and not a complete solution to your diet.

Fats and proteins can help you via your hormonal balance to stimulate satiety and curb cravings.[415]

In short, a ketogenic diet that is low in carbohydrates and high in healthy fats is ideal for setting your hormone balance on fat burning and satiety.[416]

The pleasant side effect is the prevention of modern diseases such as insulin resistance, diabetes, and cancer.[417]

Still, there is no easier way to live healthier than skipping breakfast.

Health is that simple. There is no more powerful remedy than intermittent fasting.

No other measure brings a manifold array of health benefits with minimal effort.

I want to take this opportunity to congratulate you on making it through the book. Finally, it is very science-heavy, but for a good reason.

This book contains the knowledge you need to take your health back into your own hands. That's a liberating feeling.

Implementing the knowledge into your everyday life is the only thing that offers even more freedom.

To do this, you need to actively break the outdated concept of health by making small changes to old habits.

The 30-Day Fasting Challenge gives you the tools to start today without thinking about possible mistakes.

I wish you the best in your quest to improve your health. Thank you for trusting in my work.

If you found this guide, written specifically for women, helpful, I would be delighted to receive a review on Amazon. Thank you!

Afterword

The truth about health and fitness was determined by factors we took for granted in the past.

These factors were and are strongly influenced by the market power of global food and pharma giants.

It is in our hands to create new health awareness in the information age. Today we can build the truth on a scientific basis.

All you and I have to do is open our mouths. If each of us spends a few seconds spreading this science-backed word, we can contribute to a healthier and happier world.

And the place to start is my blog.

Find free practical tips, recipes, personal support, and the latest studies on intermittent fasting on:

www.mentalfoodchain.com

References

Real Added Value for Women

[1]Fothergill E, Guo J, Howard L, Kerns JC, Knuth ND, Brychta R, Chen KY, Skarulis MC, Walter M, Walter PJ, Hall KD. Persistent metabolic adaptation 6 years after "The Biggest Loser" competition. Obesity (Silver Spring). 2016 Aug;24(8):1612-9. doi: 10.1002/oby.21538. Epub 2016 May 2. PubMed PMID: 27136388; PubMed Central PMCID: PMC4989512.

[2]Stubbs RJ, Mazlan N, Whybrow S. Carbohydrates, appetite and feeding behavior in humans. J Nutr. 2001 Oct;131(10):2775S-2781S. doi: 10.1093/jn/131.10.2775S. Review. PubMed PMID: 11584105.

Blood Sugar and Weight Loss

[3]Stárka L, Dušková M. What is a hormone?. Physiol Res. 2020 Sep 30;69(Suppl 2):S183-S185. doi: 10.33549/physiol-res.934509. Review. PubMed PMID: 33094616; PubMed Central PMCID: PMC8603735.

[4]CDC. Prevalence of Overweight, Obesity, and Extreme Obesity Among Adults: United States, Trends 1960–1962 Through 2009–2010. Atlanta, GA: Centers for Disease Control and Prevention, 2012.

[5]Lustig RH. The neuroendocrinology of childhood obesity. Pediatr Clin North Am. 2001 Aug;48(4):909-30. doi: 10.1016/s0031-3955(05)70348-5. Review. PubMed PMID: 11494643.

[6]Fildes A, Charlton J, Rudisill C, Littlejohns P, Prevost AT, Gulliford MC. Probability of an Obese Person Attaining Normal Body Weight: Cohort Study Using Electronic Health Records. Am J Public Health. 2015 Sep;105(9):e54-9. doi: 10.2105/AJPH.2015.302773. Epub 2015 Jul 16. PubMed PMID: 26180980; PubMed Central PMCID: PMC4539812.

[7]Fothergill E, Guo J, Howard L, Kerns JC, Knuth ND, Brychta R, Chen KY, Skarulis MC, Walter M, Walter PJ, Hall KD. Persistent metabolic adaptation 6 years after "The Biggest Loser" competition. Obesity (Silver Spring). 2016 Aug;24(8):1612-9. doi: 10.1002/oby.21538. Epub 2016 May 2. PubMed PMID: 27136388; PubMed Central PMCID: PMC4989512.

[8]Jensen MD, Caruso M, Heiling V, Miles JM. Insulin regulation of lipolysis in nondiabetic and IDDM subjects. Diabetes. 1989 Dec;38(12):1595-601. doi: 10.2337/diab.38.12.1595. PubMed PMID: 2573554.

[9]Meijssen S, Cabezas MC, Ballieux CG, Derksen RJ, Bilecen S, Erkelens DW. Insulin mediated inhibition of hormone sensitive lipase activity in vivo in relation to endogenous catecholamines in healthy subjects. J Clin Endocrinol Metab. 2001 Sep;86(9):4193-7. doi: 10.1210/jcem.86.9.7794. PubMed PMID: 11549649.

[10]Muretta JM, Mastick CC. How insulin regulates glucose transport in adipocytes. Vitam Horm. 2009;80:245-86. doi: 10.1016/S0083-6729(08)00610-9. Review. PubMed PMID: 19251041.

[11]Harvie MN, Pegington M, Mattson MP, Frystyk J, Dillon B, Evans G, Cuzick J, Jebb SA, Martin B, Cutler RG, Son TG, Maudsley S, Carlson OD, Egan JM, Flyvbjerg A, Howell A. The effects of intermittent or continuous energy restriction on weight loss and metabolic disease risk markers: a randomized trial in young overweight women. Int J Obes (Lond). 2011 May;35(5):714-27. doi: 10.1038/ijo.2010.171. Epub 2010 Oct 5. PubMed PMID: 20921964; PubMed Central PMCID: PMC3017674.

[12]Ali AT. Polycystic ovary syndrome and metabolic syndrome. Ceska Gynekol. 2015 Aug;80(4):279-89. Review. PubMed PMID: 26265416.

[13]Menke A, Casagrande S, Geiss L, Cowie CC. Prevalence of and Trends in Diabetes Among Adults in the United States, 1988-2012. JAMA. 2015 Sep 8;314(10):1021-9. doi: 10.1001/jama.2015.10029. PubMed PMID: 26348752.

[14]Keller U, Schnell H, Sonnenberg GE, Gerber PP, Stauffacher W. Role of glucagon in enhancing ketone body production in ketotic diabetic man. Diabetes. 1983 May;32(5):387-91. doi: 10.2337/diab.32.5.387. PubMed PMID: 6132846.

[15]Marliss EB, Aoki TT, Unger RH, Soeldner JS, Cahill GF Jr. Glucagon levels and metabolic effects in fasting man. J Clin Invest. 1970 Dec;49(12):2256-70. doi: 10.1172/JCI106445. PubMed PMID: 5480852; PubMed Central PMCID: PMC322727.

[16] Epel E, Lapidus R, McEwen B, Brownell K. Stress may add bite to appetite in women: a laboratory study of stress-induced cortisol and eating behavior. Psychoneuroendocrinology. 2001 Jan;26(1):37-49. doi: 10.1016/s0306-4530(00)00035-4. Pub-Med PMID: 11070333.

[17]Owen OE, Cahill GF Jr. Metabolic effects of exogenous glu-cocorticoids in fasted man. J Clin Invest. 1973 Oct;52(10):2596-605. doi: 10.1172/JCI107452. PubMed PMID: 4729053; PubMed Central PMCID: PMC302520.

[18]Whitworth JA, Williamson PM, Brown MA, Colman P. Hyperin-sulinemia is not a cause of cortisol-induced hypertension. Am J Hypertens. 1994 Jun;7(6):562-5. doi: 10.1093/ajh/7.6.562. PubMed PMID: 7917157.

[19]Rosmond R, Dallman MF, Björntorp P. Stress-related cortisol secretion in men: relationships with abdominal obesity and en-docrine, metabolic and hemodynamic abnormalities. J Clin En-docrinol Metab. 1998 Jun;83(6):1853-9. doi: 10.1210/jcem.83.6.4843. PubMed PMID: 9626108.

[20]Ayachi SE, Paulmyer-Lacroix O, Verdier M, Alessi MC, Dutour A, Grino M. 11beta-Hydroxysteroid dehydrogenase type 1-dri-ven cortisone reactivation regulates plasminogen activator in-hibitor type 1 in adipose tissue of obese women. J Thromb Ha-emost. 2006 Mar;4(3):621-7. doi: 10.1111/j.1538-7836.2006.01811.x. PubMed PMID: 16460444.

[21]Rask E, Walker BR, Söderberg S, Livingstone DE, Eliasson M, Johnson O, Andrew R, Olsson T. Tissue-specific changes in peripheral cortisol metabolism in obese women: increased adipose 11beta-hydroxysteroid dehydrogenase type 1 activity. J Clin Endocrinol Metab. 2002 Jul;87(7):3330-6. doi: 10.1210/jcem.87.7.8661. PubMed PMID: 12107245.

[22]Mattson MP, Longo VD, Harvie M. Impact of intermittent fasting on health and disease processes. Ageing Res Rev. 2017 Oct;39:46-58. doi: 10.1016/j.arr.2016.10.005. Epub 2016 Oct 31. Review. PubMed PMID: 27810402; PubMed Central PMCID: PMC5411330.

[23]Mozaffarian D, Rimm EB, Herrington DM. Dietary fats, carbohydrate, and progression of coronary atherosclerosis in postmenopausal women. Am J Clin Nutr. 2004 Nov;80(5):1175-84. doi: 10.1093/ajcn/80.5.1175. PubMed PMID: 15531663; PubMed Central PMCID: PMC1270002.

[24]Huang PL. A comprehensive definition for metabolic syndrome. Dis Model Mech. 2009 May-Jun;2(5-6):231-7. doi: 10.1242/dmm.001180. Review. PubMed PMID: 19407331; PubMed Central PMCID: PMC2675814.

[25]Herman ME, O'Keefe JH, Bell DSH, Schwartz SS. Insulin Therapy Increases Cardiovascular Risk in Type 2 Diabetes. Prog Cardiovasc Dis. 2017 Nov – Dec;60(3):422-434. doi: 10.1016/j.pcad.2017.09.001. Epub 2017 Sep 25. Review. PubMed PMID: 28958751.

[26]Orgel E, Mittelman SD. The links between insulin resistance, diabetes, and cancer. Curr Diab Rep. 2013 Apr;13(2):213-22. doi: 10.1007/s11892-012-0356-6. Review. PubMed PMID: 23271574; PubMed Central PMCID: PMC3595327.

[27]Ferreira LSS, Fernandes CS, Vieira MNN, De Felice FG. Insulin Resistance in Alzheimer's Disease. Front Neurosci. 2018;12:830. doi: 10.3389/fnins.2018.00830. eCollection 2018. Review. PubMed PMID: 30542257; PubMed Central PMCID: PMC6277874.

[28]Athauda D, Foltynie T. Insulin resistance and Parkinson's disease: A new target for disease modification?. Prog Neurobiol. 2016 Oct – Nov;145-146:98-120. doi: 10.1016/j.pneurobio.2016.10.001. Epub 2016 Oct 3. Review. PubMed PMID: 27713036.

[29]Reaven GM. Banting lecture 1988. Role of insulin resistance in human disease. Diabetes. 1988 Dec;37(12):1595-607. doi: 10.2337/diab.37.12.1595. Review. PubMed PMID: 3056758.

[30]Facchini FS, Hua N, Abbasi F, Reaven GM. Insulin resistance as a predictor of age-related diseases. J Clin Endocrinol Metab. 2001 Aug;86(8):3574-8. doi: 10.1210/jcem.86.8.7763. PubMed PMID: 11502781.

[31]WHO. The top 10 causes of death. Geneva: World Health Organization, 2018. Retrieved 2020 Mar 20, from https://www.who.int/news-room/fact-sheets/detail/the-top-10-causes-of-death.

[32]Wu S, Zhou K, Misra-Hebert A, Bena J, Kashyap SR. Impact of Metabolic Syndrome on Severity of COVID-19 Illness. Metab Syndr Relat Disord. 2022 May;20(4):191-198. doi: 10.1089/met.2021.0102. Epub 2022 Jan 6. PubMed PMID: 34995147.

Hunger and Satiety

[33]Mattson MP, Longo VD, Harvie M. Impact of intermittent fasting on health and disease processes. Ageing Res Rev. 2017 Oct;39:46-58. doi: 10.1016/j.arr.2016.10.005. Epub 2016 Oct 31. Review. PubMed PMID: 27810402; PubMed Central PMCID: PMC5411330.

[34] Austin J, Marks D. Hormonal regulators of appetite. Int J Pediatr Endocrinol. 2009;2009:141753. doi: 10.1155/2009/141753. Epub 2008 Dec 3. PubMed PMID: 19946401; PubMed Central PMCID: PMC2777281.

[35]Vergara RC, Jaramillo-Riveri S, Luarte A, Moënne-Loccoz C, Fuentes R, Couve A, Maldonado PE. The Energy Homeostasis Principle: Neuronal Energy Regulation Drives Local Network Dynamics Generating Behavior. Front Comput Neurosci. 2019;13:49. doi: 10.3389/fncom.2019.00049. eCollection 2019. PubMed PMID: 31396067; PubMed Central PMCID: PMC6664078.

[36]Austin J, Marks D. Hormonal regulators of appetite. Int J Pediatr Endocrinol. 2009;2009:141753. doi: 10.1155/2009/141753. Epub 2008 Dec 3. PubMed PMID: 19946401; PubMed Central PMCID: PMC2777281.

[37]Klok MD, Jakobsdottir S, Drent ML. The role of leptin and ghrelin in the regulation of food intake and body weight in humans: a review. Obes Rev. 2007 Jan;8(1):21-34. doi: 10.1111/j.1467-789X.2006.00270.x. Review. PubMed PMID: 17212793.

[38]Müller TD, Nogueiras R, Andermann ML, Andrews ZB, Anker SD, Argente J, Batterham RL, Benoit SC, Bowers CY, Broglio F, Casanueva FF, D'Alessio D, Depoortere I, Geliebter A, Ghigo E, Cole PA, Cowley M, Cummings DE, Dagher A, Diano S, Dickson SL, Diéguez C, Granata R, Grill HJ, Grove K, Habegger KM, Heppner K, Heiman ML, Holsen L, Holst B, Inui A, Jansson JO, Kirchner H, Korbonits M, Laferrère B, LeRoux CW, Lopez M, Morin S, Nakazato M, Nass R, Perez-Tilve D, Pfluger PT, Schwartz TW, Seeley RJ, Sleeman M, Sun Y, Sussel L, Tong J, Thorner MO, van der Lely AJ, van der Ploeg LH, Zigman JM, Kojima M, Kangawa K, Smith RG, Horvath T, Tschöp MH. Ghrelin. Mol Metab. 2015 Jun;4(6):437-60. doi: 10.1016/j.molmet.2015.03.005. eCollection 2015 Jun. Review. PubMed PMID: 26042199; PubMed Central PMCID: PMC4443295.

[39]Austin J, Marks D. Hormonal regulators of appetite. Int J Pediatr Endocrinol. 2009;2009:141753. doi: 10.1155/2009/141753. Epub 2008 Dec 3. PubMed PMID: 19946401; PubMed Central PMCID: PMC2777281.

[40]Klok MD, Jakobsdottir S, Drent ML. The role of leptin and ghrelin in the regulation of food intake and body weight in humans: a review. Obes Rev. 2007 Jan;8(1):21-34. doi: 10.1111/j.1467-789X.2006.00270.x. Review. PubMed PMID: 17212793.

[41]Friedman JM, Halaas JL. Leptin and the regulation of body weight in mammals. Nature. 1998 Oct 22;395(6704):763-70. doi: 10.1038/27376. Review. PubMed PMID: 9796811.

[42]Austin J, Marks D. Hormonal regulators of appetite. Int J Pediatr Endocrinol. 2009;2009:141753. doi: 10.1155/2009/141753. Epub 2008 Dec 3. PubMed PMID: 19946401; PubMed Central PMCID: PMC2777281.

[43]Myers MG Jr, Leibel RL, Seeley RJ, Schwartz MW. Obesity and leptin resistance: distinguishing cause from effect. Trends Endocrinol Metab. 2010 Nov;21(11):643-51. doi: 10.1016/j.tem.2010.08.002. Epub 2010 Sep 16. Review. PubMed PMID: 20846876; PubMed Central PMCID: PMC2967652.

[44]Martin SS, Qasim A, Reilly MP. Leptin resistance: a possible interface of inflammation and metabolism in obesity-related cardiovascular disease. J Am Coll Cardiol. 2008 Oct 7;52(15):1201-10. doi: 10.1016/j.jacc.2008.05.060. Review. PubMed PMID: 18926322; PubMed Central PMCID: PMC4556270.

[45]Lustig RH, Sen S, Soberman JE, Velasquez-Mieyer PA. Obesity, leptin resistance, and the effects of insulin reduction. Int J Obes Relat Metab Disord. 2004 Oct;28(10):1344-8. doi: 10.1038/sj.ijo.0802753. PubMed PMID: 15314628.

[46]Austin J, Marks D. Hormonal regulators of appetite. Int J Pediatr Endocrinol. 2009;2009:141753. doi: 10.1155/2009/141753. Epub 2008 Dec 3. PubMed PMID: 19946401; PubMed Central PMCID: PMC2777281.

[47]Beck B. Neuropeptide Y in normal eating and in genetic and dietary-induced obesity. Philos Trans R Soc Lond B Biol Sci. 2006 Jul 29;361(1471):1159-85. doi: 10.1098/rstb.2006.1855. Review. PubMed PMID: 16874931; PubMed Central PMCID: PMC1642692.

[48]Minor RK, Chang JW, de Cabo R. Hungry for life: How the arcuate nucleus and neuropeptide Y may play a critical role in mediating the benefits of calorie restriction. Mol Cell Endocrinol. 2009 Feb 5;299(1):79-88. doi: 10.1016/j.mce.2008.10.044. Epub 2008 Nov 11. Review. PubMed PMID: 19041366; PubMed Central PMCID: PMC2668104.

[49]Kuo LE, Kitlinska JB, Tilan JU, Li L, Baker SB, Johnson MD, Lee EW, Burnett MS, Fricke ST, Kvetnansky R, Herzog H, Zukowska Z. Neuropeptide Y acts directly in the periphery on fat tissue and mediates stress-induced obesity and metabolic syndrome. Nat Med. 2007 Jul;13(7):803-11. doi: 10.1038/nm1611. Epub 2007 Jul 1. PubMed PMID: 17603492.

[50]Reichmann F, Holzer P. Neuropeptide Y: A stressful review. Neuropeptides. 2016 Feb;55:99-109. doi: 10.1016/j.npep.2015.09.008. Epub 2015 Sep 30. Review. PubMed PMID: 26441327; PubMed Central PMCID: PMC4830398.

[51]McDonald RB, Ramsey JJ. Honoring Clive McCay and 75 years of calorie restriction research. J Nutr. 2010 Jul;140(7):1205-10. doi: 10.3945/jn.110.122804. Epub 2010 May 19. PubMed PMID: 20484554; PubMed Central PMCID: PMC2884327.

[52]Minor RK, Chang JW, de Cabo R. Hungry for life: How the arcuate nucleus and neuropeptide Y may play a critical role in mediating the benefits of calorie restriction. Mol Cell Endocrinol. 2009 Feb 5;299(1):79-88. doi: 10.1016/j.mce.2008.10.044. Epub 2008 Nov 11. Review. PubMed PMID: 19041366; PubMed Central PMCID: PMC2668104.

[53]Wu Y, He H, Cheng Z, Bai Y, Ma X. The Role of Neuropeptide Y and Peptide YY in the Development of Obesity via Gut-brain Axis. Curr Protein Pept Sci. 2019;20(7):750-758. doi: 10.2174/1389203720666190125105401. Review. PubMed PMID: 30678628.

[54]Pironi L, Stanghellini V, Miglioli M, Corinaldesi R, De Giorgio R, Ruggeri E, Tosetti C, Poggioli G, Morselli Labate AM, Monetti N. Fat-induced ileal brake in humans: a dose-dependent phenomenon correlated to the plasma levels of peptide YY. Gastroenterology. 1993 Sep;105(3):733-9. doi: 10.1016/0016-5085(93)90890-o. PubMed PMID: 8359644.

[55]Wu Y, He H, Cheng Z, Bai Y, Ma X. The Role of Neuropeptide Y and Peptide YY in the Development of Obesity via Gut-brain Axis. Curr Protein Pept Sci. 2019;20(7):750-758. doi: 10.2174/1389203720666190125105401. Review. PubMed PMID: 30678628.

[56]Zwirska-Korczala K, Konturek SJ, Sodowski M, Wylezol M, Kuka D, Sowa P, Adamczyk-Sowa M, Kukla M, Berdowska A, Rehfeld JF, Bielanski W, Brzozowski T. Basal and postprandial plasma levels of PYY, ghrelin, cholecystokinin, gastrin and insulin in women with moderate and morbid obesity and metabolic syndrome. J Physiol Pharmacol. 2007 Mar;58 Suppl 1:13-35. PubMed PMID: 17443025.

[57]Zouhal H, Sellami M, Saeidi A, Slimani M, Abbassi-Daloii A, Khodamoradi A, El Hage R, Hackney AC, Ben Abderrahman A. Effect of physical exercise and training on gastrointestinal hormones in populations with different weight statuses. Nutr Rev. 2019 Jul 1;77(7):455-477. doi: 10.1093/nutrit/nuz005. Review. PubMed PMID: 31125091.

[58]Cahill F, Shea JL, Randell E, Vasdev S, Sun G. Serum peptide YY in response to short-term overfeeding in young men. Am J Clin Nutr. 2011 Apr;93(4):741-7. doi: 10.3945/ajcn.110.003624. Epub 2011 Feb 2. PubMed PMID: 21289220.

[59]Müller TD, Finan B, Bloom SR, D'Alessio D, Drucker DJ, Flatt PR, Fritsche A, Gribble F, Grill HJ, Habener JF, Holst JJ, Langhans W, Meier JJ, Nauck MA, Perez-Tilve D, Pocai A, Reimann F, Sandoval DA, Schwartz TW, Seeley RJ, Stemmer K, Tang-Christensen M, Woods SC, DiMarchi RD, Tschöp MH. Glucagon-like peptide 1 (GLP-1). Mol Metab. 2019 Dec;30:72-130. doi: 10.1016/j.molmet.2019.09.010. Epub 2019 Sep 30. Review. PubMed PMID: 31767182; PubMed Central PMCID: PMC6812410.

[60]Zhang F, Tong Y, Su N, Li Y, Tang L, Huang L, Tong N. Weight loss effect of glucagon-like peptide-1 mimetics on obese/overweight adults without diabetes: A systematic review and meta-analysis of randomized controlled trials. J Diabetes. 2015 May;7(3):329-39. doi: 10.1111/1753-0407.12198. Epub 2014 Sep 10. Review. PubMed PMID: 25043423.

[61]Morínigo R, Moizé V, Musri M, Lacy AM, Navarro S, Marín JL, Delgado S, Casamitjana R, Vidal J. Glucagon-like peptide-1, peptide YY, hunger, and satiety after gastric bypass surgery in morbidly obese subjects. J Clin Endocrinol Metab. 2006 May;91(5):1735-40. doi: 10.1210/jc.2005-0904. Epub 2006 Feb 14. PubMed PMID: 16478824.

[62]Müller TD, Finan B, Bloom SR, D'Alessio D, Drucker DJ, Flatt PR, Fritsche A, Gribble F, Grill HJ, Habener JF, Holst JJ, Langhans W, Meier JJ, Nauck MA, Perez-Tilve D, Pocai A, Reimann F, Sandoval DA, Schwartz TW, Seeley RJ, Stemmer K, Tang-Christensen M, Woods SC, DiMarchi RD, Tschöp MH. Glucagon-like peptide 1 (GLP-1). Mol Metab. 2019 Dec;30:72-130. doi: 10.1016/j.molmet.2019.09.010. Epub 2019 Sep 30. Review. PubMed PMID: 31767182; PubMed Central PMCID: PMC6812410.

[63]Anandhakrishnan A, Korbonits M. Glucagon-like peptide 1 in the pathophysiology and pharmacotherapy of clinical obesity. World J Diabetes. 2016 Dec 15;7(20):572-598. doi: 10.4239/wjd.v7.i20.572. Review. PubMed PMID: 28031776; PubMed Central PMCID: PMC5155232.

[64]Stinson SE, Jonsson AE, Lund MAV, Frithioff-Bøjsøe C, Aas Holm L, Pedersen O, Ängquist L, Sørensen TIA, Holst JJ, Christiansen M, Holm JC, Hartmann B, Hansen T. Fasting Plasma GLP-1 Is Associated With Overweight/Obesity and Cardiometabolic Risk Factors in Children and Adolescents. J Clin Endocrinol Metab. 2021 May 13;106(6):1718-1727. doi: 10.1210/clinem/dgab098. PubMed PMID: 33596309; PubMed Central PMCID: PMC8118577.

[65]Gibbs J, Young RC, Smith GP. Cholecystokinin elicits satiety in rats with open gastric fistulas. Nature. 1973 Oct 12;245(5424):323-5. doi: 10.1038/245323a0. PubMed PMID: 4586439.

[66]Konturek JW, Konturek SJ, Kwiecień N, Bielański W, Pawlik T, Rembiasz K, Domschke W. Leptin in the control of gastric secretion and gut hormones in humans infected with Helicobacter pylori. Scand J Gastroenterol. 2001 Nov;36(11):1148-54. doi: 10.1080/00365520152584761. PubMed PMID: 11686213.

[67]Peters JH, Simasko SM, Ritter RC. Modulation of vagal afferent excitation and reduction of food intake by leptin and cholecystokinin. Physiol Behav. 2006 Nov 30;89(4):477-85. doi: 10.1016/j.physbeh.2006.06.017. Epub 2006 Jul 26. Review. PubMed PMID: 16872644.

[68]Liddle RA, Goldfine ID, Rosen MS, Taplitz RA, Williams JA. Cholecystokinin bioactivity in human plasma. Molecular forms, responses to feeding, and relationship to gallbladder contraction. J Clin Invest. 1985 Apr;75(4):1144-52. doi: 10.1172/JCI111809. PubMed PMID: 2580857; PubMed Central PMCID: PMC425438.

[69]Okonkwo O, Zezoff D, Adeyinka A. Biochemistry, Cholecystokinin. [Updated 2021 May 9]. In: StatPearls [Internet]. Treasure Island (FL): StatPearls Publishing; 2022 Jan-. Available from: https://www.ncbi.nlm.nih.gov/books/NBK534204/

[70]Dockray GJ. Cholecystokinin. Curr Opin Endocrinol Diabetes Obes. 2012 Feb;19(1):8-12. doi: 10.1097/MED.0b013e32834eb77d. Review. PubMed PMID: 22157397.

[71]Lieverse RJ, Jansen JB, Masclee AA, Lamers CB. Satiety effects of a physiological dose of cholecystokinin in humans. Gut. 1995 Feb;36(2):176-9. doi: 10.1136/gut.36.2.176. PubMed PMID: 7883212; PubMed Central PMCID: PMC1382399.

Sexuality and Fertility

[72]Cawthon CR, de La Serre CB. The critical role of CCK in the regulation of food intake and diet-induced obesity. Peptides. 2021 Apr;138:170492. doi: 10.1016/j.peptides.2020.170492. Epub 2021 Jan 8. Review. PubMed PMID: 33422646.

[73]Lovejoy JC. The influence of sex hormones on obesity across the female life span. J Womens Health. 1998 Dec;7(10):1247-56. doi: 10.1089/jwh.1998.7.1247. Review. PubMed PMID: 9929857.

[74]Tyagi V, Scordo M, Yoon RS, Liporace FA, Greene LW. Revisiting the role of testosterone: Are we missing something?. Rev Urol. 2017;19(1):16-24. doi: 10.3909/riu0716. PubMed PMID: 28522926; PubMed Central PMCID: PMC5434832.

[75]De Pergola G. The adipose tissue metabolism: role of testosterone and dehydroepiandrosterone. Int J Obes Relat Metab Disord. 2000 Jun;24 Suppl 2:S59-63. doi: 10.1038/sj.ijo.0801280. Review. PubMed PMID: 10997611.

[76]Rebuffé-Scrive M, Mårin P, Björntorp P. Effect of testosterone on abdominal adipose tissue in men. Int J Obes. 1991 Nov;15(11):791-5. PubMed PMID: 1778664.

[77]Swerdloff RS, Ng CM. Gynecomastia: Etiology, Diagnosis, and Treatment. [Updated 2019 Jul 7]. In: Feingold KR, Anawalt B, Boyce A, et al., editors. Endotext [Internet]. South Dartmouth (MA): MDText.com, Inc.; 2000-. Available from: https://www.ncbi.nlm.nih.gov/books/NBK279105/

[78]Daka B, Rosen T, Jansson PA, Råstam L, Larsson CA, Lindblad U. Inverse association between serum insulin and sex hormone-binding globulin in a population survey in Sweden. Endocr Connect. 2013 Mar 1;2(1):18-22. doi: 10.1530/EC-12-0057. Print 2013 Mar 1. PubMed PMID: 23781314; PubMed Central PMCID: PMC3680959.

[79]Mihm M, Gangooly S, Muttukrishna S. The normal menstrual cycle in women. Anim Reprod Sci. 2011 Apr;124(3-4):229-36. doi: 10.1016/j.anireprosci.2010.08.030. Epub 2010 Sep 3. Review. PubMed PMID: 20869180.

[80]Reed BG, Carr BR. The Normal Menstrual Cycle and the Control of Ovulation. 2000;. Review. PubMed PMID: 25905282.

[81]Reed BG, Carr BR. The Normal Menstrual Cycle and the Control of Ovulation. 2000;. Review. PubMed PMID: 25905282.

[82]Reed BG, Carr BR. The Normal Menstrual Cycle and the Control of Ovulation. 2000;. Review. PubMed PMID: 25905282.

[83]Reed BG, Carr BR. The Normal Menstrual Cycle and the Control of Ovulation. 2000;. Review. PubMed PMID: 25905282.

[84]Reed BG, Carr BR. The Normal Menstrual Cycle and the Control of Ovulation. 2000;. Review. PubMed PMID: 25905282.

What Is Fasting?

[85]BUCHINGER O Sr. [40 Years of fasting therapy]. Hippokrates. 1959 Mar 31;30(6):246-8. PubMed PMID: 13653601.

[86]Levine B, Klionsky DJ. Autophagy wins the 2016 Nobel Prize in Physiology or Medicine: Breakthroughs in baker's yeast fuel advances in biomedical research. Proc Natl Acad Sci U S A. 2017 Jan 10;114(2):201-205. doi: 10.1073/pnas.1619876114. Epub 2016 Dec 30. PubMed PMID: 28039434; PubMed Central PMCID: PMC5240711.

[87]Jiao J, Demontis F. Skeletal muscle autophagy and its role in sarcopenia and organismal aging. Curr Opin Pharmacol. 2017 Jun;34:1-6. doi: 10.1016/j.coph.2017.03.009. Epub 2017 Apr 10. Review. PubMed PMID: 28407519.

[88]Nakamura S, Yoshimori T. Autophagy and Longevity. Mol Cells. 2018 Jan 31;41(1):65-72. doi: 10.14348/molcells.2018.2333. Epub 2018 Jan 23. Review. PubMed PMID: 29370695; PubMed Central PMCID: PMC5792715.

[89]Yang JS, Lu CC, Kuo SC, Hsu YM, Tsai SC, Chen SY, Chen YT, Lin YJ, Huang YC, Chen CJ, Lin WD, Liao WL, Lin WY, Liu YH, Sheu JC, Tsai FJ. Autophagy and its link to type II diabetes mellitus. Biomedicine (Taipei). 2017 Jun;7(2):8. doi: 10.1051/bmdcn/2017070201. Epub 2017 Jun 14. PubMed PMID: 28612706; PubMed Central PMCID: PMC5479440.

[90]Puigserver A, Wicker C, Gaucher C. [Molecular aspects of the adaptation of pancreatic and intestinal enzymes to dietary regimens]. Reprod Nutr Dev. 1985;25(4B):787-801. PubMed PMID: 2417292.

Top 10 Fasting Myths Debunked by Science

[91]Stubbs RJ, Mazlan N, Whybrow S. Carbohydrates, appetite and feeding behavior in humans. J Nutr. 2001 Oct;131(10):2775S-2781S. doi: 10.1093/jn/131.10.2775S. Review. PubMed PMID: 11584105.

[92]Cameron JD, Cyr MJ, Doucet E. Increased meal frequency does not promote greater weight loss in subjects who were prescribed an 8-week equi-energetic energy-restricted diet. Br J Nutr. 2010 Apr;103(8):1098-101. doi: 10.1017/S0007114509992984. Epub 2009 Nov 30. PubMed PMID: 19943985.

[93]Kong LC, Wuillemin PH, Bastard JP, Sokolovska N, Gougis S, Fellahi S, Darakhshan F, Bonnefont-Rousselot D, Bittar R, Doré J, Zucker JD, Clément K, Rizkalla S. Insulin resistance and inflammation predict kinetic body weight changes in response to dietary weight loss and maintenance in overweight and obese subjects by using a Bayesian network approach. Am J Clin Nutr. 2013 Dec;98(6):1385-94. doi: 10.3945/ajcn.113.058099. Epub 2013 Oct 30. PubMed PMID: 24172304.

[94]Meijssen S, Cabezas MC, Ballieux CG, Derksen RJ, Bilecen S, Erkelens DW. Insulin mediated inhibition of hormone sensitive lipase activity in vivo in relation to endogenous catecholamines in healthy subjects. J Clin Endocrinol Metab. 2001 Sep;86(9):4193-7. doi: 10.1210/jcem.86.9.7794. PubMed PMID: 11549649.

[95]Fothergill E, Guo J, Howard L, Kerns JC, Knuth ND, Brychta R, Chen KY, Skarulis MC, Walter M, Walter PJ, Hall KD. Persistent metabolic adaptation 6 years after "The Biggest Loser" competition. Obesity (Silver Spring). 2016 Aug;24(8):1612-9. doi: 10.1002/oby.21538. Epub 2016 May 2. PubMed PMID: 27136388; PubMed Central PMCID: PMC4989512.

[96]Meijssen S, Cabezas MC, Ballieux CG, Derksen RJ, Bilecen S, Erkelens DW. Insulin mediated inhibition of hormone sensitive lipase activity in vivo in relation to endogenous catecholamines in healthy subjects. J Clin Endocrinol Metab. 2001 Sep;86(9):4193-7. doi: 10.1210/jcem.86.9.7794. PubMed PMID: 11549649.

[97]Ho KY, Veldhuis JD, Johnson ML, Furlanetto R, Evans WS, Alberti KG, Thorner MO. Fasting enhances growth hormone secretion and amplifies the complex rhythms of growth hormone secretion in man. J Clin Invest. 1988 Apr;81(4):968-75. doi: 10.1172/JCI113450. PubMed PMID: 3127426; PubMed Central PMCID: PMC329619.

[98]DRENICK EJ, SWENDSEID ME, BLAHD WH, TUTTLE SG. PROLONGED STARVATION AS TREATMENT FOR SEVERE OBESITY. JAMA. 1964 Jan 11;187:100-5. doi: 10.1001/jama.1964.03060150024006. PubMed PMID: 14066725.

[99]Zauner C, Schneeweiss B, Kranz A, Madl C, Ratheiser K, Kramer L, Roth E, Schneider B, Lenz K. Resting energy expenditure in short-term starvation is increased as a result of an increase in serum norepinephrine. Am J Clin Nutr. 2000 Jun;71(6):1511-5. doi: 10.1093/ajcn/71.6.1511. PubMed PMID: 10837292.

[100]Patel JN, Coppack SW, Goldstein DS, Miles JM, Eisenhofer G. Norepinephrine spillover from human adipose tissue before and after a 72-hour fast. J Clin Endocrinol Metab. 2002 Jul;87(7):3373-7. doi: 10.1210/jcem.87.7.8695. PubMed PMID: 12107252.

[101]Ho KY, Veldhuis JD, Johnson ML, Furlanetto R, Evans WS, Alberti KG, Thorner MO. Fasting enhances growth hormone secretion and amplifies the complex rhythms of growth hormone secretion in man. J Clin Invest. 1988 Apr;81(4):968-75. doi: 10.1172/JCI113450. PubMed PMID: 3127426; PubMed Central PMCID: PMC329619.

[102]Jiao J, Demontis F. Skeletal muscle autophagy and its role in sarcopenia and organismal aging. Curr Opin Pharmacol. 2017 Jun;34:1-6. doi: 10.1016/j.coph.2017.03.009. Epub 2017 Apr 10. Review. PubMed PMID: 28407519.

[103]Paoli A, Bosco G, Camporesi EM, Mangar D. Ketosis, ketogenic diet and food intake control: a complex relationship. Front Psychol. 2015;6:27. doi: 10.3389/fpsyg.2015.00027. eCollection 2015. Review. PubMed PMID: 25698989; PubMed Central PMCID: PMC4313585.

[104]Rudman D, Feller AG, Nagraj HS, Gergans GA, Lalitha PY, Goldberg AF, Schlenker RA, Cohn L, Rudman IW, Mattson DE. Effects of human growth hormone in men over 60 years old. N Engl J Med. 1990 Jul 5;323(1):1-6. doi: 10.1056/NEJM199007053230101. PubMed PMID: 2355952.

[105]Besson A, Salemi S, Gallati S, Jenal A, Horn R, Mullis PS, Mullis PE. Reduced longevity in untreated patients with isolated growth hormone deficiency. J Clin Endocrinol Metab. 2003 Aug;88(8):3664-7. doi: 10.1210/jc.2002-021938. PubMed PMID: 12915652.

[106]Arnal MA, Mosoni L, Boirie Y, Houlier ML, Morin L, Verdier E, Ritz P, Antoine JM, Prugnaud J, Beaufrère B, Mirand PP. Protein feeding pattern does not affect protein retention in young women. J Nutr. 2000 Jul;130(7):1700-4. doi: 10.1093/jn/130.7.1700. PubMed PMID: 10867039.

[107]Arnal MA, Mosoni L, Boirie Y, Houlier ML, Morin L, Verdier E, Ritz P, Antoine JM, Prugnaud J, Beaufrère B, Mirand PP. Protein pulse feeding improves protein retention in elderly women. Am J Clin Nutr. 1999 Jun;69(6):1202-8. doi: 10.1093/ajcn/69.6.1202. PubMed PMID: 10357740.

[108]Merimee TJ, Tyson JE. Stabilization of plasma glucose during fasting; Normal variations in two separate studies. N Engl J Med. 1974 Dec 12;291(24):1275-8. doi: 10.1056/NEJM197412122912404. PubMed PMID: 4431434.

[109]Anton SD, Moehl K, Donahoo WT, Marosi K, Lee SA, Mainous AG 3rd, Leeuwenburgh C, Mattson MP. Flipping the Metabolic Switch: Understanding and Applying the Health Benefits of Fasting. Obesity (Silver Spring). 2018 Feb;26(2):254-268. doi: 10.1002/oby.22065. Epub 2017 Oct 31. Review. PubMed PMID: 29086496; PubMed Central PMCID: PMC5783752.

[110]Melkonian EA, Asuka E, Schury MP. Physiology, Gluconeogenesis. 2021 Jan;. Review. PubMed PMID: 31082163.

[111]Hallböök T, Ji S, Maudsley S, Martin B. The effects of the ketogenic diet on behavior and cognition. Epilepsy Res. 2012 Jul;100(3):304-9. doi: 10.1016/j.eplepsyres.2011.04.017. Epub 2011 Aug 27. Review. PubMed PMID: 21872440; PubMed Central PMCID: PMC4112040.

[112]LaManna JC, Salem N, Puchowicz M, Erokwu B, Koppaka S, Flask C, Lee Z. Ketones suppress brain glucose consumption. Adv Exp Med Biol. 2009;645:301-6. doi: 10.1007/978-0-387-85998-9_45. PubMed PMID: 19227486; PubMed Central PMCID: PMC2874681.

[113]Cannataro R, Caroleo MC, Fazio A, La Torre C, Plastina P, Gallelli L, Lauria G, Cione E. Ketogenic Diet and microRNAs Linked to Antioxidant Biochemical Homeostasis. Antioxidants (Basel). 2019 Aug 2;8(8). doi: 10.3390/antiox8080269. PubMed PMID: 31382449; PubMed Central PMCID: PMC6719224.

[114]Kim DH, Park MH, Ha S, Bang EJ, Lee Y, Lee AK, Lee J, Yu BP, Chung HY. Anti-inflammatory action of β-hydroxybutyrate via modulation of PGC-1α and FoxO1, mimicking calorie restriction. Aging (Albany NY). 2019 Feb 27;11(4):1283-1304. doi: 10.18632/aging.101838. PubMed PMID: 30811347; PubMed Central PMCID: PMC6402511.

[115]Stewart WK, Fleming LW. Features of a successful therapeutic fast of 382 days' duration. Postgrad Med J. 1973 Mar;49(569):203-9. doi: 10.1136/pgmj.49.569.203. PubMed PMID: 4803438; PubMed Central PMCID: PMC2495396.

[116]Levine B, Klionsky DJ. Autophagy wins the 2016 Nobel Prize in Physiology or Medicine: Breakthroughs in baker's yeast fuel advances in biomedical research. Proc Natl Acad Sci U S A. 2017 Jan 10;114(2):201-205. doi: 10.1073/pnas.1619876114. Epub 2016 Dec 30. PubMed PMID: 28039434; PubMed Central PMCID: PMC5240711.

[117]Johnstone AM, Faber P, Gibney ER, Elia M, Horgan G, Golden BE, Stubbs RJ. Effect of an acute fast on energy compensation and feeding behaviour in lean men and women. Int J Obes Relat Metab Disord. 2002 Dec;26(12):1623-8. doi: 10.1038/sj.ijo.0802151. PubMed PMID: 12461679.

[118]Natalucci G, Riedl S, Gleiss A, Zidek T, Frisch H. Spontaneous 24-h ghrelin secretion pattern in fasting subjects: maintenance of a meal-related pattern. Eur J Endocrinol. 2005 Jun;152(6):845-50. doi: 10.1530/eje.1.01919. PubMed PMID: 15941923.

[119]Wüst S, Wolf J, Hellhammer DH, Federenko I, Schommer N, Kirschbaum C. The cortisol awakening response – normal values and confounds. Noise Health. 2000;2(7):79-88. PubMed PMID: 12689474.

[120]Dhurandhar EJ, Dawson J, Alcorn A, Larsen LH, Thomas EA, Cardel M, Bourland AC, Astrup A, St-Onge MP, Hill JO, Apovian CM, Shikany JM, Allison DB. The effectiveness of breakfast recommendations on weight loss: a randomized controlled trial. Am J Clin Nutr. 2014 Aug;100(2):507-13. doi: 10.3945/ajcn.114.089573. Epub 2014 Jun 4. PubMed PMID: 24898236; PubMed Central PMCID: PMC4095657.

[121]Heilbronn LK, Smith SR, Martin CK, Anton SD, Ravussin E. Alternate-day fasting in nonobese subjects: effects on body weight, body composition, and energy metabolism. Am J Clin Nutr. 2005 Jan;81(1):69-73. doi: 10.1093/ajcn/81.1.69. PubMed PMID: 15640462.

[122]Cho Y, Hong N, Kim KW, Cho SJ, Lee M, Lee YH, Lee YH, Kang ES, Cha BS, Lee BW. The Effectiveness of Intermittent Fasting to Reduce Body Mass Index and Glucose Metabolism: A Systematic Review and Meta-Analysis. J Clin Med. 2019 Oct 9;8(10). doi: 10.3390/jcm8101645. PubMed PMID: 31601019; PubMed Central PMCID: PMC6832593.

Is Intermittent Fasting Suitable for Women?

[123]Meczekalski B, Podfigurna-Stopa A, Warenik-Szymankiewicz A, Genazzani AR. Functional hypothalamic amenorrhea: current view on neuroendocrine aberrations. Gynecol Endocrinol. 2008 Jan;24(1):4-11. doi: 10.1080/09513590701807381. Review. PubMed PMID: 18224538.

[124]Meczekalski B, Katulski K, Czyzyk A, Podfigurna-Stopa A, Maciejewska-Jeske M. Functional hypothalamic amenorrhea and its influence on women's health. J Endocrinol Invest. 2014 Nov;37(11):1049-56. doi: 10.1007/s40618-014-0169-3. Epub 2014 Sep 9. Review. PubMed PMID: 25201001; PubMed Central PMCID: PMC4207953.

[125]Kumar S, Kaur G. Intermittent fasting dietary restriction regimen negatively influences reproduction in young rats: a study of hypothalamo-hypophysial-gonadal axis. PLoS One. 2013;8(1):e52416. doi: 10.1371/journal.pone.0052416. Epub 2013 Jan 29. PubMed PMID: 23382817; PubMed Central PMCID: PMC3558496.

[126]Martin B, Pearson M, Kebejian L, Golden E, Keselman A, Bender M, Carlson O, Egan J, Ladenheim B, Cadet JL, Becker KG, Wood W, Duffy K, Vinayakumar P, Maudsley S, Mattson MP. Sex-dependent metabolic, neuroendocrine, and cognitive responses to dietary energy restriction and excess. Endocrinology. 2007 Sep;148(9):4318-33. doi: 10.1210/en.2007-0161. Epub 2007 Jun 14. PubMed PMID: 17569758; PubMed Central PMCID: PMC2622430.

[127]Trepanowski JF, Kroeger CM, Barnosky A, Klempel MC, Bhutani S, Hoddy KK, Gabel K, Freels S, Rigdon J, Rood J, Ravussin E, Varady KA. Effect of Alternate-Day Fasting on Weight Loss, Weight Maintenance, and Cardioprotection Among Metabolically Healthy Obese Adults: A Randomized Clinical Trial. JAMA Intern Med. 2017 Jul 1;177(7):930-938. doi: 10.1001/jamainternmed.2017.0936. PubMed PMID: 28459931; PubMed Central PMCID: PMC5680777.

[128]Martin B, Pearson M, Kebejian L, Golden E, Keselman A, Bender M, Carlson O, Egan J, Ladenheim B, Cadet JL, Becker KG, Wood W, Duffy K, Vinayakumar P, Maudsley S, Mattson MP. Sex-dependent metabolic, neuroendocrine, and cognitive responses to dietary energy restriction and excess. Endocrinology. 2007 Sep;148(9):4318-33. doi: 10.1210/en.2007-0161. Epub 2007 Jun 14. PubMed PMID: 17569758; PubMed Central PMCID: PMC2622430.

How Women Fast Safely

[129]Yang JS, Lu CC, Kuo SC, Hsu YM, Tsai SC, Chen SY, Chen YT, Lin YJ, Huang YC, Chen CJ, Lin WD, Liao WL, Lin WY, Liu YH, Sheu JC, Tsai FJ. Autophagy and its link to type II diabetes melli-tus. Biomedicine (Taipei). 2017 Jun;7(2):8. doi: 10.1051/bmdcn/2017070201. Epub 2017 Jun 14. PubMed PMID: 28612706; PubMed Central PMCID: PMC5479440.

[130]Meczekalski B, Katulski K, Czyzyk A, Podfigurna-Stopa A, Maciejewska-Jeske M. Functional hypothalamic amenorrhea and its influence on women's health. J Endocrinol Invest. 2014 Nov;37(11):1049-56. doi: 10.1007/s40618-014-0169-3. Epub 2014 Sep 9. Review. PubMed PMID: 25201001; PubMed Central PMCID: PMC4207953.

[131]Natalucci G, Riedl S, Gleiss A, Zidek T, Frisch H. Spontaneous 24-h ghrelin secretion pattern in fasting subjects: maintenance of a meal-related pattern. Eur J Endocrinol. 2005 Jun;152(6):845-50. doi: 10.1530/eje.1.01919. PubMed PMID: 15941923.

[132]Meczekalski B, Katulski K, Czyzyk A, Podfigurna-Stopa A, Maciejewska-Jeske M. Functional hypothalamic amenorrhea and its influence on women's health. J Endocrinol Invest. 2014 Nov;37(11):1049-56. doi: 10.1007/s40618-014-0169-3. Epub 2014 Sep 9. Review. PubMed PMID: 25201001; PubMed Central PMCID: PMC4207953.

Why 16 Hours of Fasting Work

[133]Gill S, Panda S. A Smartphone App Reveals Erratic Diurnal Eating Patterns in Humans that Can Be Modulated for Health Benefits. Cell Metab. 2015 Nov 3;22(5):789-98. doi: 10.1016/j.cmet.2015.09.005. Epub 2015 Sep 24. PubMed PMID: 26411343; PubMed Central PMCID: PMC4635036.

[134]Levine B, Klionsky DJ. Autophagy wins the 2016 Nobel Prize in Physiology or Medicine: Breakthroughs in baker's yeast fuel advances in biomedical research. Proc Natl Acad Sci U S A. 2017 Jan 10;114(2):201-205. doi: 10.1073/pnas.1619876114. Epub 2016 Dec 30. PubMed PMID: 28039434; PubMed Central PMCID: PMC5240711.

[135]Yang JS, Lu CC, Kuo SC, Hsu YM, Tsai SC, Chen SY, Chen YT, Lin YJ, Huang YC, Chen CJ, Lin WD, Liao WL, Lin WY, Liu YH, Sheu JC, Tsai FJ. Autophagy and its link to type II diabetes mellitus. Biomedicine (Taipei). 2017 Jun;7(2):8. doi: 10.1051/bmdcn/2017070201. Epub 2017 Jun 14. PubMed PMID: 28612706; PubMed Central PMCID: PMC5479440.

[136]Meijssen S, Cabezas MC, Ballieux CG, Derksen RJ, Bilecen S, Erkelens DW. Insulin mediated inhibition of hormone sensitive lipase activity in vivo in relation to endogenous catecholamines in healthy subjects. J Clin Endocrinol Metab. 2001 Sep;86(9):4193-7. doi: 10.1210/jcem.86.9.7794. PubMed PMID: 11549649.

[137]Albalat A, Saera-Vila A, Capilla E, Gutiérrez J, Pérez-Sánchez J, Navarro I. Insulin regulation of lipoprotein lipase (LPL) activity and expression in gilthead sea bream (Sparus aurata). Comp Biochem Physiol B Biochem Mol Biol. 2007 Oct;148(2):151-9. doi: 10.1016/j.cbpb.2007.05.004. Epub 2007 May 18. PubMed PMID: 17600746.

[138]Kong LC, Wuillemin PH, Bastard JP, Sokolovska N, Gougis S, Fellahi S, Darakhshan F, Bonnefont-Rousselot D, Bittar R, Doré J, Zucker JD, Clément K, Rizkalla S. Insulin resistance and inflammation predict kinetic body weight changes in response to dietary weight loss and maintenance in overweight and obese subjects by using a Bayesian network approach. Am J Clin Nutr. 2013 Dec;98(6):1385-94. doi: 10.3945/ajcn.113.058099. Epub 2013 Oct 30. PubMed PMID: 24172304.

[139]Holman RR, Thorne KI, Farmer AJ, Davies MJ, Keenan JF, Paul S, Levy JC. Addition of biphasic, prandial, or basal insulin to oral therapy in type 2 diabetes. N Engl J Med. 2007 Oct 25;357(17):1716-30. doi: 10.1056/NEJMoa075392. Epub 2007 Sep 21. PubMed PMID: 17890232.

[140]Shah PK, Mudaliar S, Chang AR, Aroda V, Andre M, Burke P, Henry RR. Effects of intensive insulin therapy alone and in combination with pioglitazone on body weight, composition, distribution and liver fat content in patients with type 2 diabetes. Diabetes Obes Metab. 2011 Jun;13(6):505-10. doi: 10.1111/j.1463-1326.2011.01370.x. PubMed PMID: 21272186; PubMed Central PMCID: PMC3580155.

[141]Heilbronn LK, Smith SR, Martin CK, Anton SD, Ravussin E. Alternate-day fasting in nonobese subjects: effects on body weight, body composition, and energy metabolism. Am J Clin Nutr. 2005 Jan;81(1):69-73. doi: 10.1093/ajcn/81.1.69. PubMed PMID: 15640462.

[142]Courchesne-Loyer A, Croteau E, Castellano CA, St-Pierre V, Hennebelle M, Cunnane SC. Inverse relationship between brain glucose and ketone metabolism in adults during short-term moderate dietary ketosis: A dual tracer quantitative positron emission tomography study. J Cereb Blood Flow Metab. 2017 Jul;37(7):2485-2493. doi: 10.1177/0271678X16669366. Epub 2016 Jan 1. PubMed PMID: 27629100; PubMed Central PMCID: PMC5531346.

[143]Prasanth MI, Sivamaruthi BS, Chaiyasut C, Tencomnao T. A Review of the Role of Green Tea (Camellia sinensis) in Antiphotoaging, Stress Resistance, Neuroprotection, and Autophagy. Nutrients. 2019 Feb 23;11(2). doi: 10.3390/nu11020474. Review. PubMed PMID: 30813433; PubMed Central PMCID: PMC6412948.

[144]Yang JS, Lu CC, Kuo SC, Hsu YM, Tsai SC, Chen SY, Chen YT, Lin YJ, Huang YC, Chen CJ, Lin WD, Liao WL, Lin WY, Liu YH, Sheu JC, Tsai FJ. Autophagy and its link to type II diabetes mellitus. Biomedicine (Taipei). 2017 Jun;7(2):8. doi: 10.1051/bmdcn/2017070201. Epub 2017 Jun 14. PubMed PMID: 28612706; PubMed Central PMCID: PMC5479440.

[145]Sasaki Y, Ikeda Y, Iwabayashi M, Akasaki Y, Ohishi M. The Impact of Autophagy on Cardiovascular Senescence and Diseases. Int Heart J. 2017 Oct 21;58(5):666-673. doi: 10.1536/ihj.17-246. Epub 2017 Sep 30. Review. PubMed PMID: 28966332.

[146]Nair PM, Khawale PG. Role of therapeutic fasting in women's health: An overview. J Midlife Health. 2016 Apr-Jun;7(2):61-4. doi: 10.4103/0976-7800.185325. Review. PubMed PMID: 27499591; PubMed Central PMCID: PMC4960941.

[147]Raefsky SM, Mattson MP. Adaptive responses of neuronal mitochondria to bioenergetic challenges: Roles in neuroplasticity and disease resistance. Free Radic Biol Med. 2017 Jan;102:203-216. doi: 10.1016/j.freeradbiomed.2016.11.045. Epub 2016 Nov 29. Review. PubMed PMID: 27908782; PubMed Central PMCID: PMC5209274.

[148]Levine B, Klionsky DJ. Autophagy wins the 2016 Nobel Prize in Physiology or Medicine: Breakthroughs in baker's yeast fuel advances in biomedical research. Proc Natl Acad Sci U S A. 2017 Jan 10;114(2):201-205. doi: 10.1073/pnas.1619876114. Epub 2016 Dec 30. PubMed PMID: 28039434; PubMed Central PMCID: PMC5240711.

Health Benefits for Women

[149]Bagheriya M, Butler AE, Barreto GE, Sahebkar A. The effect of fasting or calorie restriction on autophagy induction: A review of the literature. Ageing Res Rev. 2018 Nov;47:183-197. doi: 10.1016/j.arr.2018.08.004. Epub 2018 Aug 30. Review. PubMed PMID: 30172870.

[150]Raefsky SM, Mattson MP. Adaptive responses of neuronal mitochondria to bioenergetic challenges: Roles in neuroplasticity and disease resistance. Free Radic Biol Med. 2017 Jan;102:203-216. doi: 10.1016/j.freeradbiomed.2016.11.045. Epub 2016 Nov 29. Review. PubMed PMID: 27908782; PubMed Central PMCID: PMC5209274.

[151]Jiao J, Demontis F. Skeletal muscle autophagy and its role in sarcopenia and organismal aging. Curr Opin Pharmacol. 2017 Jun;34:1-6. doi: 10.1016/j.coph.2017.03.009. Epub 2017 Apr 10. Review. PubMed PMID: 28407519.

[152]Sasaki Y, Ikeda Y, Iwabayashi M, Akasaki Y, Ohishi M. The Impact of Autophagy on Cardiovascular Senescence and Diseases. Int Heart J. 2017 Oct 21;58(5):666-673. doi: 10.1536/ihj.17-246. Epub 2017 Sep 30. Review. PubMed PMID: 28966332.

[153]Nakamura S, Yoshimori T. Autophagy and Longevity. Mol Cells. 2018 Jan 31;41(1):65-72. doi: 10.14348/molcells.2018.2333. Epub 2018 Jan 23. Review. PubMed PMID: 29370695; PubMed Central PMCID: PMC5792715.

[154]Yang JS, Lu CC, Kuo SC, Hsu YM, Tsai SC, Chen SY, Chen YT, Lin YJ, Huang YC, Chen CJ, Lin WD, Liao WL, Lin WY, Liu YH, Sheu JC, Tsai FJ. Autophagy and its link to type II diabetes mellitus. Biomedicine (Taipei). 2017 Jun;7(2):8. doi: 10.1051/bmdcn/2017070201. Epub 2017 Jun 14. PubMed PMID: 28612706; PubMed Central PMCID: PMC5479440.

[155]Sasaki Y, Ikeda Y, Iwabayashi M, Akasaki Y, Ohishi M. The Impact of Autophagy on Cardiovascular Senescence and Diseases. Int Heart J. 2017 Oct 21;58(5):666-673. doi: 10.1536/ihj.17-246. Epub 2017 Sep 30. Review. PubMed PMID: 28966332.

[156]Gelino S, Hansen M. Autophagy – An Emerging Anti-Aging Mechanism. J Clin Exp Pathol. 2012 Jul 12;Suppl 4. doi: 10.4172/2161-0681.s4-006. PubMed PMID: 23750326; Pub-Med Central PMCID: PMC3674854.

[157]Nakamura S, Yoshimori T. Autophagy and Longevity. Mol Cells. 2018 Jan 31;41(1):65-72. doi: 10.14348/molcells.2018.2333. Epub 2018 Jan 23. Review. PubMed PMID: 29370695; PubMed Central PMCID: PMC5792715.

[158]Catterson JH, Khericha M, Dyson MC, Vincent AJ, Callard R, Haveron SM, Rajasingam A, Ahmad M, Partridge L. Short-Term, Intermittent Fasting Induces Long-Lasting Gut Health and TOR-Independent Lifespan Extension. Curr Biol. 2018 Jun 4;28(11):1714-1724.e4. doi: 10.1016/j.cub.2018.04.015. Epub 2018 May 17. PubMed PMID: 29779873; PubMed Central PMCID: PMC5988561.

[159]Diot A, Morten K, Poulton J. Mitophagy plays a central role in mitochondrial ageing. Mamm Genome. 2016 Aug;27(7-8):381-95. doi: 10.1007/s00335-016-9651-x. Epub 2016 Jun 28. Review. PubMed PMID: 27352213; PubMed Central PMCID: PMC4935730.

[160]Gill S, Panda S. A Smartphone App Reveals Erratic Diurnal Eating Patterns in Humans that Can Be Modulated for Health Benefits. Cell Metab. 2015 Nov 3;22(5):789-98. doi: 10.1016/j.cmet.2015.09.005. Epub 2015 Sep 24. PubMed PMID: 26411343; PubMed Central PMCID: PMC4635036.

[161]Li X, Chen H, Guan Y, Li X, Lei L, Liu J, Yin L, Liu G, Wang Z. Acetic acid activates the AMP-activated protein kinase signaling pathway to regulate lipid metabolism in bovine hepatocytes. PLoS One. 2013;8(7):e67880. doi: 10.1371/journal.pone.0067880. Print 2013. PubMed PMID: 23861826; Pub-Med Central PMCID: PMC3701595.

[162]Raefsky SM, Mattson MP. Adaptive responses of neuronal mitochondria to bioenergetic challenges: Roles in neuroplasticity and disease resistance. Free Radic Biol Med. 2017 Jan;102:203-216. doi: 10.1016/j.freeradbiomed.2016.11.045. Epub 2016 Nov 29. Review. PubMed PMID: 27908782; PubMed Central PMCID: PMC5209274.

[163]Witte AV, Fobker M, Gellner R, Knecht S, Flöel A. Caloric restriction improves memory in elderly humans. Proc Natl Acad Sci U S A. 2009 Jan 27;106(4):1255-60. doi: 10.1073/pnas.0808587106. Epub 2009 Jan 26. PubMed PMID: 19171901; PubMed Central PMCID: PMC2633586.

[164]Lieberman HR, Caruso CM, Niro PJ, Adam GE, Kellogg MD, Nindl BC, Kramer FM. A double-blind, placebo-controlled test of 2 d of calorie deprivation: effects on cognition, activity, sleep, and interstitial glucose concentrations. Am J Clin Nutr. 2008 Sep;88(3):667-76. doi: 10.1093/ajcn/88.3.667. PubMed PMID: 18779282.

[165]Fond G, Macgregor A, Leboyer M, Michalsen A. Fasting in mood disorders: neurobiology and effectiveness. A review of the literature. Psychiatry Res. 2013 Oct 30;209(3):253-8. doi: 10.1016/j.psychres.2012.12.018. Epub 2013 Jan 15. Review. PubMed PMID: 23332541.

[166]DRENICK EJ, SWENDSEID ME, BLAHD WH, TUTTLE SG. PROLONGED STARVATION AS TREATMENT FOR SEVERE OBESITY. JAMA. 1964 Jan 11;187:100-5. doi: 10.1001/jama.1964.03060150024006. PubMed PMID: 14066725.

[167]Ho KY, Veldhuis JD, Johnson ML, Furlanetto R, Evans WS, Alberti KG, Thorner MO. Fasting enhances growth hormone secretion and amplifies the complex rhythms of growth hormone secretion in man. J Clin Invest. 1988 Apr;81(4):968-75. doi: 10.1172/JCI113450. PubMed PMID: 3127426; PubMed Central PMCID: PMC329619.

[168]Zauner C, Schneeweiss B, Kranz A, Madl C, Ratheiser K, Kramer L, Roth E, Schneider B, Lenz K. Resting energy expenditure in short-term starvation is increased as a result of an increase in serum norepinephrine. Am J Clin Nutr. 2000 Jun;71(6):1511-5. doi: 10.1093/ajcn/71.6.1511. PubMed PMID: 10837292.

[169]Rudman D, Feller AG, Nagraj HS, Gergans GA, Lalitha PY, Goldberg AF, Schlenker RA, Cohn L, Rudman IW, Mattson DE. Effects of human growth hormone in men over 60 years old. N Engl J Med. 1990 Jul 5;323(1):1-6. doi: 10.1056/NEJM199007053230101. PubMed PMID: 2355952.

[170]Ho KY, Veldhuis JD, Johnson ML, Furlanetto R, Evans WS, Alberti KG, Thorner MO. Fasting enhances growth hormone secretion and amplifies the complex rhythms of growth hormone secretion in man. J Clin Invest. 1988 Apr;81(4):968-75. doi: 10.1172/JCI113450. PubMed PMID: 3127426; PubMed Central PMCID: PMC329619.

[171]Paoli A, Bosco G, Camporesi EM, Mangar D. Ketosis, ketogenic diet and food intake control: a complex relationship. Front Psychol. 2015;6:27. doi: 10.3389/fpsyg.2015.00027. eCollection 2015. Review. PubMed PMID: 25698989; PubMed Central PMCID: PMC4313585.

[172]Hallböök T, Ji S, Maudsley S, Martin B. The effects of the ketogenic diet on behavior and cognition. Epilepsy Res. 2012 Jul;100(3):304-9. doi: 10.1016/j.eplepsyres.2011.04.017. Epub 2011 Aug 27. Review. PubMed PMID: 21872440; PubMed Central PMCID: PMC4112040.

[173]Catenacci VA, Pan Z, Ostendorf D, Brannon S, Gozansky WS, Mattson MP, Martin B, MacLean PS, Melanson EL, Troy Donahoo W. A randomized pilot study comparing zero-calorie alternate-day fasting to daily caloric restriction in adults with obesity. Obesity (Silver Spring). 2016 Sep;24(9):1874-83. doi: 10.1002/oby.21581. PubMed PMID: 27569118; PubMed Central PMCID: PMC5042570.

174Bray GA, Jablonski KA, Fujimoto WY, Barrett-Connor E, Haffner S, Hanson RL, Hill JO, Hubbard V, Kriska A, Stamm E, Pi-Sunyer FX. Relation of central adiposity and body mass index to the development of diabetes in the Diabetes Prevention Program. Am J Clin Nutr. 2008 May;87(5):1212-8. doi: 10.1093/ajcn/87.5.1212. PubMed PMID: 18469241; PubMed Central PMCID: PMC2517222.

175Jackson IM, McKiddie MT, Buchanan KD. Effect of fasting on glucose and insulin metabolism of obese patients. Lancet. 1969 Feb 8;1(7589):285-7. doi: 10.1016/s0140-6736(69)91039-3. PubMed PMID: 4178981.

176Catenacci VA, Pan Z, Ostendorf D, Brannon S, Gozansky WS, Mattson MP, Martin B, MacLean PS, Melanson EL, Troy Donahoo W. A randomized pilot study comparing zero-calorie alternate-day fasting to daily caloric restriction in adults with obesity. Obesity (Silver Spring). 2016 Sep;24(9):1874-83. doi: 10.1002/oby.21581. PubMed PMID: 27569118; PubMed Central PMCID: PMC5042570.

177Halberg N, Henriksen M, Söderhamn N, Stallknecht B, Ploug T, Schjerling P, Dela F. Effect of intermittent fasting and refeeding on insulin action in healthy men. J Appl Physiol (1985). 2005 Dec;99(6):2128-36. doi: 10.1152/japplphysiol.00683.2005. Epub 2005 Jul 28. PubMed PMID: 16051710.

178Ali AT. Polycystic ovary syndrome and metabolic syndrome. Ceska Gynekol. 2015 Aug;80(4):279-89. Review. PubMed PMID: 26265416.

179Nair PM, Khawale PG. Role of therapeutic fasting in women's health: An overview. J Midlife Health. 2016 Apr-Jun;7(2):61-4. doi: 10.4103/0976-7800.185325. Review. PubMed PMID: 27499591; PubMed Central PMCID: PMC4960941.

[180]Mihaylova MM, Cheng CW, Cao AQ, Tripathi S, Mana MD, Bauer-Rowe KE, Abu-Remaileh M, Clavain L, Erdemir A, Lewis CA, Freinkman E, Dickey AS, La Spada AR, Huang Y, Bell GW, Deshpande V, Carmeliet P, Katajisto P, Sabatini DM, Yilmaz ÖH. Fasting Activates Fatty Acid Oxidation to Enhance Intestinal Stem Cell Function during Homeostasis and Aging. Cell Stem Cell. 2018 May 3;22(5):769-778.e4. doi: 10.1016/j.stem.2018.04.001. PubMed PMID: 29727683; PubMed Central PMCID: PMC5940005.

[181]Catterson JH, Khericha M, Dyson MC, Vincent AJ, Callard R, Haveron SM, Rajasingam A, Ahmad M, Partridge L. Short-Term, Intermittent Fasting Induces Long-Lasting Gut Health and TOR-Independent Lifespan Extension. Curr Biol. 2018 Jun 4;28(11):1714-1724.e4. doi: 10.1016/j.cub.2018.04.015. Epub 2018 May 17. PubMed PMID: 29779873; PubMed Central PMCID: PMC5988561.

[182]Mihaylova MM, Cheng CW, Cao AQ, Tripathi S, Mana MD, Bauer-Rowe KE, Abu-Remaileh M, Clavain L, Erdemir A, Lewis CA, Freinkman E, Dickey AS, La Spada AR, Huang Y, Bell GW, Deshpande V, Carmeliet P, Katajisto P, Sabatini DM, Yilmaz ÖH. Fasting Activates Fatty Acid Oxidation to Enhance Intestinal Stem Cell Function during Homeostasis and Aging. Cell Stem Cell. 2018 May 3;22(5):769-778.e4. doi: 10.1016/j.stem.2018.04.001. PubMed PMID: 29727683; PubMed Central PMCID: PMC5940005.

[183]Cheng CW, Adams GB, Perin L, Wei M, Zhou X, Lam BS, Da Sacco S, Mirisola M, Quinn DI, Dorff TB, Kopchick JJ, Longo VD. Prolonged fasting reduces IGF-1/PKA to promote hematopoietic-stem-cell-based regeneration and reverse immunosuppression. Cell Stem Cell. 2014 Jun 5;14(6):810-23. doi: 10.1016/j.stem.2014.04.014. PubMed PMID: 24905167; PubMed Central PMCID: PMC4102383.

184Patterson RE, Laughlin GA, LaCroix AZ, Hartman SJ, Natarajan L, Senger CM, Martínez ME, Villaseñor A, Sears DD, Marinac CR, Gallo LC. Intermittent Fasting and Human Metabolic Health. J Acad Nutr Diet. 2015 Aug;115(8):1203-12. doi: 10.1016/j.jand.2015.02.018. Epub 2015 Apr 6. PubMed PMID: 25857868; PubMed Central PMCID: PMC4516560.

185Mattson MP, Longo VD, Harvie M. Impact of intermittent fasting on health and disease processes. Ageing Res Rev. 2017 Oct;39:46-58. doi: 10.1016/j.arr.2016.10.005. Epub 2016 Oct 31. Review. PubMed PMID: 27810402; PubMed Central PMCID: PMC5411330.

186Panda S, Hogenesch JB, Kay SA. Circadian rhythms from flies to human. Nature. 2002 May 16;417(6886):329-35. doi: 10.1038/417329a. Review. PubMed PMID: 12015613.

187Patterson RE, Sears DD. Metabolic Effects of Intermittent Fasting. Annu Rev Nutr. 2017 Aug 21;37:371-393. doi: 10.1146/annurev-nutr-071816-064634. Epub 2017 Jul 17. Review. PubMed PMID: 28715993.

188Hatori M, Vollmers C, Zarrinpar A, DiTacchio L, Bushong EA, Gill S, Leblanc M, Chaix A, Joens M, Fitzpatrick JA, Ellisman MH, Panda S. Time-restricted feeding without reducing caloric intake prevents metabolic diseases in mice fed a high-fat diet. Cell Metab. 2012 Jun 6;15(6):848-60. doi: 10.1016/j.cmet.2012.04.019. Epub 2012 May 17. PubMed PMID: 22608008; PubMed Central PMCID: PMC3491655.

189Savvidis C, Koutsilieris M. Circadian rhythm disruption in cancer biology. Mol Med. 2012 Dec 6;18:1249-60. doi: 10.2119/molmed.2012.00077. Review. PubMed PMID: 22811066; PubMed Central PMCID: PMC3521792.

190Scheer FA, Hilton MF, Mantzoros CS, Shea SA. Adverse metabolic and cardiovascular consequences of circadian misalignment. Proc Natl Acad Sci U S A. 2009 Mar 17;106(11):4453-8. doi: 10.1073/pnas.0808180106. Epub 2009 Mar 2. PubMed PMID: 19255424; PubMed Central PMCID: PMC2657421.

How Intermittent Fasting Helps with PMS

191Mishra S, Elliott H, Marwaha R. Premenstrual Dysphoric Disorder. 2022 Jan;. PubMed PMID: 30335340.

192A DM, K S, A D, Sattar K. Epidemiology of Premenstrual Syndrome (PMS)-A Systematic Review and Meta-Analysis Study. J Clin Diagn Res. 2014 Feb;8(2):106-9. doi: 10.7860/JCDR/2014/8024.4021. Epub 2014 Feb 3. PubMed PMID: 24701496; PubMed Central PMCID: PMC3972521.

193Fatemi M, Allahdadian M, Bahadorani M. Comparison of serum level of some trace elements and vitamin D between patients with premenstrual syndrome and normal controls: A cross-sectional study. Int J Reprod Biomed. 2019 Sep;17(9):647-652. doi: 10.18502/ijrm.v17i9.5100. eCollection 2019 Sep. PubMed PMID: 31646259; PubMed Central PMCID: PMC6804325.

194Hoddy KK, Kroeger CM, Trepanowski JF, Barnosky AR, Bhutani S, Varady KA. Safety of alternate day fasting and effect on disordered eating behaviors. Nutr J. 2015 May 6;14:44. doi: 10.1186/s12937-015-0029-9. PubMed PMID: 25943396; PubMed Central PMCID: PMC4424827.

[195]Jamshed H, Beyl RA, Della Manna DL, Yang ES, Ravussin E, Peterson CM. Early Time-Restricted Feeding Improves 24-Hour Glucose Levels and Affects Markers of the Circadian Clock, Aging, and Autophagy in Humans. Nutrients. 2019 May 30;11(6). doi: 10.3390/nu11061234. PubMed PMID: 31151228; PubMed Central PMCID: PMC6627766.

[196]Witte AV, Fobker M, Gellner R, Knecht S, Flöel A. Caloric restriction improves memory in elderly humans. Proc Natl Acad Sci U S A. 2009 Jan 27;106(4):1255-60. doi: 10.1073/pnas.0808587106. Epub 2009 Jan 26. PubMed PMID: 19171901; PubMed Central PMCID: PMC2633586.

[197]Daka B, Rosen T, Jansson PA, Råstam L, Larsson CA, Lindblad U. Inverse association between serum insulin and sex hormone-binding globulin in a population survey in Sweden. Endocr Connect. 2013 Mar 1;2(1):18-22. doi: 10.1530/EC-12-0057. Print 2013 Mar 1. PubMed PMID: 23781314; PubMed Central PMCID: PMC3680959.

[198]Hara Y, Waters EM, McEwen BS, Morrison JH. Estrogen Effects on Cognitive and Synaptic Health Over the Lifecourse. Physiol Rev. 2015 Jul;95(3):785-807. doi: 10.1152/physrev.00036.2014. Review. PubMed PMID: 26109339; PubMed Central PMCID: PMC4491541.[199]Gudipally PR, Sharma GK. Premenstrual Syndrome. 2022 Jan;. PubMed PMID: 32809533.

[199]Harvie MN, Pegington M, Mattson MP, Frystyk J, Dillon B, Evans G, Cuzick J, Jebb SA, Martin B, Cutler RG, Son TG, Maudsley S, Carlson OD, Egan JM, Flyvbjerg A, Howell A. The effects of intermittent or continuous energy restriction on weight loss and metabolic disease risk markers: a randomized trial in young overweight women. Int J Obes (Lond). 2011 May;35(5):714-27. doi: 10.1038/ijo.2010.171. Epub 2010 Oct 5. PubMed PMID: 20921964; PubMed Central PMCID: PMC3017674.

[200]Triantafillou S, Saeb S, Lattie EG, Mohr DC, Kording KP. Relationship Between Sleep Quality and Mood: Ecological Momentary Assessment Study. JMIR Ment Health. 2019 Mar 27;6(3):e12613. doi: 10.2196/12613. PubMed PMID: 30916663; PubMed Central PMCID: PMC6456824.

[201]Michalsen A, Schlegel F, Rodenbeck A, Lüdtke R, Huether G, Teschler H, Dobos GJ. Effects of short-term modified fasting on sleep patterns and daytime vigilance in non-obese subjects: results of a pilot study. Ann Nutr Metab. 2003;47(5):194-200. doi: 10.1159/000070485. PubMed PMID: 12748412.

[202]Lewis P, Oster H, Korf HW, Foster RG, Erren TC. Food as a circadian time cue - evidence from human studies. Nat Rev Endocrinol. 2020 Apr;16(4):213-223. doi: 10.1038/s41574-020-0318-z. Epub 2020 Feb 13. Review. PubMed PMID: 32055029.

[203]Michalsen A, Schlegel F, Rodenbeck A, Lüdtke R, Huether G, Teschler H, Dobos GJ. Effects of short-term modified fasting on sleep patterns and daytime vigilance in non-obese subjects: results of a pilot study. Ann Nutr Metab. 2003;47(5):194-200. doi: 10.1159/000070485. PubMed PMID: 12748412.

[204]Longo VD, Mattson MP. Fasting: molecular mechanisms and clinical applications. Cell Metab. 2014 Feb 4;19(2):181-92. doi: 10.1016/j.cmet.2013.12.008. Epub 2014 Jan 16. Review. PubMed PMID: 24440038; PubMed Central PMCID: PMC3946160.

[205]Jamshed H, Beyl RA, Della Manna DL, Yang ES, Ravussin E, Peterson CM. Early Time-Restricted Feeding Improves 24-Hour Glucose Levels and Affects Markers of the Circadian Clock, Aging, and Autophagy in Humans. Nutrients. 2019 May 30;11(6). doi: 10.3390/nu11061234. PubMed PMID: 31151228; PubMed Central PMCID: PMC6627766.

[206]Gold EB, Wells C, Rasor MO. The Association of Inflammation with Premenstrual Symptoms. J Womens Health (Larchmt). 2016 Sep;25(9):865-74. doi: 10.1089/jwh.2015.5529. Epub 2016 May 2. PubMed PMID: 27135720; PubMed Central PMCID: PMC5311461.

[207]Jordan S, Tung N, Casanova-Acebes M, Chang C, Cantoni C, Zhang D, Wirtz TH, Naik S, Rose SA, Brocker CN, Gainullina A, Hornburg D, Horng S, Maier BB, Cravedi P, LeRoith D, Gonzalez FJ, Meissner F, Ochando J, Rahman A, Chipuk JE, Artyomov MN, Frenette PS, Piccio L, Berres ML, Gallagher EJ, Merad M. Dietary Intake Regulates the Circulating Inflammatory Monocyte Pool. Cell. 2019 Aug 22;178(5):1102-1114.e17. doi: 10.1016/j.cell.2019.07.050. PubMed PMID: 31442403; PubMed Central PMCID: PMC7357241.

[208]Faris MA, Kacimi S, Al-Kurd RA, Fararjeh MA, Bustanji YK, Mohammad MK, Salem ML. Intermittent fasting during Ramadan attenuates proinflammatory cytokines and immune cells in healthy subjects. Nutr Res. 2012 Dec;32(12):947-55. doi: 10.1016/j.nutres.2012.06.021. Epub 2012 Oct 4. PubMed PMID: 23244540.

Intermittent Fasting and Pregnancy

[209]Glazier JD, Hayes DJL, Hussain S, D'Souza SW, Whitcombe J, Heazell AEP, Ashton N. The effect of Ramadan fasting during pregnancy on perinatal outcomes: a systematic review and meta-analysis. BMC Pregnancy Childbirth. 2018 Oct 25;18(1):421. doi: 10.1186/s12884-018-2048-y. PubMed PMID: 30359228; PubMed Central PMCID: PMC6202808.

[210]Petherick ES, Tuffnell D, Wright J. Experiences and outcomes of maternal Ramadan fasting during pregnancy: results from a sub-cohort of the Born in Bradford birth cohort study. BMC Pregnancy Childbirth. 2014 Sep 26;14:335. doi: 10.1186/1471-2393-14-335. PubMed PMID: 25261183; PubMed Central PMCID: PMC4261761.

[211]Safari K, Piro TJ, Ahmad HM. Perspectives and pregnancy outcomes of maternal Ramadan fasting in the second trimester of pregnancy. BMC Pregnancy Childbirth. 2019 Apr 15;19(1):128. doi: 10.1186/s12884-019-2275-x. PubMed PMID: 30987614; PubMed Central PMCID: PMC6466666.

[212]Felig P, Lynch V. Starvation in human pregnancy: hypoglycemia, hypoinsulinemia, and hyperketonemia. Science. 1970 Nov 27;170(3961):990-2. doi: 10.1126/science.170.3961.990. PubMed PMID: 5529067.

[213]Zauner C, Schneeweiss B, Kranz A, Madl C, Ratheiser K, Kramer L, Roth E, Schneider B, Lenz K. Resting energy expenditure in short-term starvation is increased as a result of an increase in serum norepinephrine. Am J Clin Nutr. 2000 Jun;71(6):1511-5. doi: 10.1093/ajcn/71.6.1511. PubMed PMID: 10837292.

[214]Mirghani HM, Weerasinghe SD, Smith JR, Ezimokhai M. The effect of intermittent maternal fasting on human fetal breathing movements. J Obstet Gynaecol. 2004 Sep;24(6):635-7. doi: 10.1080/01443610400007844. PubMed PMID: 16147601.

[215]Petherick ES, Tuffnell D, Wright J. Experiences and outcomes of maternal Ramadan fasting during pregnancy: results from a sub-cohort of the Born in Bradford birth cohort study. BMC Pregnancy Childbirth. 2014 Sep 26;14:335. doi: 10.1186/1471-2393-14-335. PubMed PMID: 25261183; PubMed Central PMCID: PMC4261761.

[216]Garzon S, Cacciato PM, Certelli C, Salvaggio C, Magliarditi M, Rizzo G. Iron Deficiency Anemia in Pregnancy: Novel Approaches for an Old Problem. Oman Med J. 2020 Sep;35(5):e166. doi: 10.5001/omj.2020.108. eCollection 2020 Sep. Review. PubMed PMID: 32953141; PubMed Central PMCID: PMC7477519.

[217]Nair PM, Khawale PG. Role of therapeutic fasting in women's health: An overview. J Midlife Health. 2016 Apr-Jun;7(2):61-4. doi: 10.4103/0976-7800.185325. Review. PubMed PMID: 27499591; PubMed Central PMCID: PMC4960941.

[218]Ali AT. Polycystic ovary syndrome and metabolic syndrome. Ceska Gynekol. 2015 Aug;80(4):279-89. Review. PubMed PMID: 26265416.

[219]Fica S, Albu A, Constantin M, Dobri GA. Insulin resistance and fertility in polycystic ovary syndrome. J Med Life. 2008 Oct-Dec;1(4):415-22. Review. PubMed PMID: 20108521; PubMed Central PMCID: PMC3018970.

[220]Nasiri-Amiri F, Sepidarkish M, Shirvani MA, Habibipour P, Tabari NSM. The effect of exercise on the prevention of gestational diabetes in obese and overweight pregnant women: a systematic review and meta-analysis. Diabetol Metab Syndr. 2019;11:72. doi: 10.1186/s13098-019-0470-6. eCollection 2019. Review. PubMed PMID: 31467594; PubMed Central PMCID: PMC6712661.

[221]Owe KM, Nystad W, Stigum H, Vangen S, Bø K. Exercise during pregnancy and risk of cesarean delivery in nulliparous women: a large population-based cohort study. Am J Obstet Gynecol. 2016 Dec;215(6):791.e1-791.e13. doi: 10.1016/j.ajog.2016.08.014. Epub 2016 Aug 23. PubMed PMID: 27555317.

[222]Varady KA, Bhutani S, Church EC, Klempel MC. Short-term modified alternate-day fasting: a novel dietary strategy for weight loss and cardioprotection in obese adults. Am J Clin Nutr. 2009 Nov;90(5):1138-43. doi: 10.3945/ajcn.2009.28380. Epub 2009 Sep 30. PubMed PMID: 19793855.

[223]Watkins E, Serpell L. The Psychological Effects of Short-Term Fasting in Healthy Women. Front Nutr. 2016;3:27. doi: 10.3389/fnut.2016.00027. eCollection 2016. PubMed PMID: 27597946; PubMed Central PMCID: PMC4992682.

Clean vs. Dirty Fasting

[224]Levine B, Klionsky DJ. Autophagy wins the 2016 Nobel Prize in Physiology or Medicine: Breakthroughs in baker's yeast fuel advances in biomedical research. Proc Natl Acad Sci U S A. 2017 Jan 10;114(2):201-205. doi: 10.1073/pnas.1619876114. Epub 2016 Dec 30. PubMed PMID: 28039434; PubMed Central PMCID: PMC5240711.

[225]The Self NutritionData method and system [Internet]. New York: Condé Nast; c2018 [cited 2021 Jan 29]. Available from: https://nutritiondata.self.com/facts/dairy-and-egg-products/51/2.

[226]The Self NutritionData method and system [Internet]. New York: Condé Nast; c2018 [cited 2021 Jan 29]. Available from: https://nutritiondata.self.com/facts/dairy-and-egg-products/69/2.

[227]The Self NutritionData method and system [Internet]. New York: Condé Nast; c2018 [cited 2021 Jan 29]. Available from: https://nutritiondata.self.com/facts/custom/278488/2.

[228]The Self NutritionData method and system [Internet]. New York: Condé Nast; c2018 [cited 2021 Jan 29]. Available from: https://nutritiondata.self.com/facts/custom/2244512/2.

229The Self NutritionData method and system [Internet]. New York: Condé Nast; c2018 [cited 2021 Jan 29]. Available from: https://nutritiondata.self.com/facts/custom/2522911/2.

230The Self NutritionData method and system [Internet]. New York: Condé Nast; c2018 [cited 2021 Jan 29]. Available from: https://nutritiondata.self.com/facts/recipe/2768812/2.

231The Self NutritionData method and system [Internet]. New York: Condé Nast; c2018 [cited 2021 Jan 29]. Available from: https://nutritiondata.self.com/facts/fruits-and-fruit-juices/1938/2.

232Department of Agriculture, Agricultural Research Service [Internet]. FoodData Central, c2019. [cited 2022 Jun 01]. Available from: https://fdc.nal.usda.gov/fdc-app.html#/food-details/1627869/nutrients.

233Department of Agriculture, Agricultural Research Service [Internet]. FoodData Central, c2019. [cited 2022 Jun 01]. Available from: https://fdc.nal.usda.gov/fdc-app.html#/food-details/170257/nutrients.

234Department of Agriculture, Agricultural Research Service [Internet]. FoodData Central, c2019. [cited 2022 Jun 01]. Available from: https://fdc.nal.usda.gov/fdc-app.html#/food-details/170679/nutrients.

235The Self NutritionData method and system [Internet]. New York: Condé Nast; c2018 [cited 2021 Jan 29]. Available from: https://nutritiondata.self.com/facts/custom/757544/1.

236The Self NutritionData method and system [Internet]. New York: Condé Nast; c2018 [cited 2021 Jan 29]. Available from: https://nutritiondata.self.com/facts/sweets/5568/2.

237The Self NutritionData method and system [Internet]. New York: Condé Nast; c2018 [cited 2021 Jan 29]. Available from: https://nutritiondata.self.com/facts/sweets/7607/2.

238Nuttall FQ, Gannon MC. Plasma glucose and insulin response to macronutrients in nondiabetic and NIDDM subjects. Diabetes Care. 1991 Sep;14(9):824-38. doi: 10.2337/diacare.14.9.824. Review. PubMed PMID: 1959475.

[239]Anton SD, Martin CK, Han H, Coulon S, Cefalu WT, Geiselman P, Williamson DA. Effects of stevia, aspartame, and sucrose on food intake, satiety, and postprandial glucose and insulin levels. Appetite. 2010 Aug;55(1):37-43. doi: 10.1016/j.appet.2010.03.009. Epub 2010 Mar 18. PubMed PMID: 20303371; PubMed Central PMCID: PMC2900484.

[240]Liang Y, Steinbach G, Maier V, Pfeiffer EF. The effect of artificial sweetener on insulin secretion. 1. The effect of acesulfame K on insulin secretion in the rat (studies in vivo). Horm Metab Res. 1987 Jun;19(6):233-8. doi: 10.1055/s-2007-1011788. PubMed PMID: 2887500.

[241]Pepino MY, Tiemann CD, Patterson BW, Wice BM, Klein S. Sucralose affects glycemic and hormonal responses to an oral glucose load. Diabetes Care. 2013 Sep;36(9):2530-5. doi: 10.2337/dc12-2221. Epub 2013 Apr 30. PubMed PMID: 23633524; PubMed Central PMCID: PMC3747933.

[242]Jeppesen PB, Gregersen S, Poulsen CR, Hermansen K. Stevioside acts directly on pancreatic beta cells to secrete insulin: actions independent of cyclic adenosine monophosphate and adenosine triphosphate-sensitive K+-channel activity. Metabolism. 2000 Feb;49(2):208-14. doi: 10.1016/s0026-0495(00)91325-8. PubMed PMID: 10690946.

[243]Zhou Y, Zheng Y, Ebersole J, Huang CF. Insulin secretion stimulating effects of mogroside V and fruit extract of luo han kuo (Siraitia grosvenori Swingle) fruit extract.. Yao Xue Xue Bao. 2009 Nov;44(11):1252-7. PubMed PMID: 21351724.

[244]The Self NutritionData method and system [Internet]. New York: Condé Nast; c2018 [cited 2021 Jan 29]. Available from: https://nutritiondata.self.com/facts/dairy-and-egg-products/51/2.

[245]The Self NutritionData method and system [Internet]. New York: Condé Nast; c2018 [cited 2021 Jan 29]. Available from: https://nutritiondata.self.com/facts/custom/2244512/2.

[246]The Self NutritionData method and system [Internet]. New York: Condé Nast; c2018 [cited 2021 Jan 29]. Available from: https://nutritiondata.self.com/facts/custom/2522911/2.

[247]The Self NutritionData method and system [Internet]. New York: Condé Nast; c2018 [cited 2021 Jan 29]. Available from: https://nutritiondata.self.com/facts/recipe/2768812/2.

[248]The Self NutritionData method and system [Internet]. New York: Condé Nast; c2018 [cited 2021 Jan 29]. Available from: https://nutritiondata.self.com/facts/dairy-and-egg-products/69/2.

[249]Department of Agriculture, Agricultural Research Service [Internet]. FoodData Central, c2019. [cited 2022 Jun 01]. Available from: https://fdc.nal.usda.gov/fdc-app.html#/food-details/1627869/nutrients.

[250]Department of Agriculture, Agricultural Research Service [Internet]. FoodData Central, c2019. [cited 2022 Jun 01]. Available from: https://fdc.nal.usda.gov/fdc-app.html#/food-details/170257/nutrients.

[251]Department of Agriculture, Agricultural Research Service [Internet]. FoodData Central, c2019. [cited 2022 Jun 01]. Available from: https://fdc.nal.usda.gov/fdc-app.html#/food-details/170679/nutrients.

[252]The Self NutritionData method and system [Internet]. New York: Condé Nast; c2018 [cited 2021 Jan 29]. Available from: https://nutritiondata.self.com/facts/custom/757544/1.

[253]The Self NutritionData method and system [Internet]. New York: Condé Nast; c2018 [cited 2021 Jan 29]. Available from: https://nutritiondata.self.com/facts/sweets/5568/2.

[254]Yang Q. Gain weight by "going diet?" Artificial sweeteners and the neurobiology of sugar cravings: Neuroscience 2010. Yale J Biol Med. 2010 Jun;83(2):101-8. PMID: 20589192; PMCID: PMC2892765.

Top 5 Intermittent Fasting Mistakes

[255]Park J, Kwock CK, Yang YJ. The Effect of the Sodium to Potassium Ratio on Hypertension Prevalence: A Propensity Score Matching Approach. Nutrients. 2016 Aug 6;8(8). doi: 10.3390/nu8080482. PubMed PMID: 27509520; PubMed Central PMCID: PMC4997395.

[256]Noh HM, Park SY, Lee HS, Oh HY, Paek YJ, Song HJ, Park KH. Association between High Blood Pressure and Intakes of Sodium and Potassium among Korean Adults: Korean National Health and Nutrition Examination Survey, 2007-2012. J Acad Nutr Diet. 2015 Dec;115(12):1950-7. doi: 10.1016/j.jand.2015.04.021. Epub 2015 Jun 27. PubMed PMID: 26129945.

[257]Fung J. The Obesity Code: Unlocking the Secrets of Weight Loss. Vancouver: Greystone Books, 2016.

[258]Sakuyama H, Katoh M, Wakabayashi H, Zulli A, Kruzliak P, Uehara Y. Influence of gestational salt restriction in fetal growth and in development of diseases in adulthood. J Biomed Sci. 2016 Jan 20;23:12. doi: 10.1186/s12929-016-0233-8. Review. PubMed PMID: 26787358; PubMed Central PMCID: PMC4719732.

[259]Ho KY, Veldhuis JD, Johnson ML, Furlanetto R, Evans WS, Alberti KG, Thorner MO. Fasting enhances growth hormone secretion and amplifies the complex rhythms of growth hormone secretion in man. J Clin Invest. 1988 Apr;81(4):968-75. doi: 10.1172/JCI113450. PubMed PMID: 3127426; PubMed Central PMCID: PMC329619.

[260]Fung J. The Obesity Code: Unlocking the Secrets of Weight Loss. Vancouver: Greystone Books, 2016.

Intermittent Fasting and Working Out

[261]Lustig RH. The neuroendocrinology of childhood obesity. Pediatr Clin North Am. 2001 Aug;48(4):909-30. doi: 10.1016/s0031-3955(05)70348-5. Review. PubMed PMID: 11494643.

[262]Melanson EL, Keadle SK, Donnelly JE, Braun B, King NA. Resistance to exercise-induced weight loss: compensatory behavioral adaptations. Med Sci Sports Exerc. 2013 Aug;45(8):1600-9. doi: 10.1249/MSS.0b013e31828ba942. Review. PubMed PMID: 23470300; PubMed Central PMCID: PMC3696411.

[263]Achten J, Jeukendrup AE. Optimizing fat oxidation through exercise and diet. Nutrition. 2004 Jul-Aug;20(7-8):716-27. doi: 10.1016/j.nut.2004.04.005. Review. PubMed PMID: 15212756.

[264]Horowitz JF, Mora-Rodriguez R, Byerley LO, Coyle EF. Lipolytic suppression following carbohydrate ingestion limits fat oxidation during exercise. Am J Physiol. 1997 Oct;273(4):E768-75. doi: 10.1152/ajpendo.1997.273.4.E768. PubMed PMID: 9357807.

[265]Jansen D, De Strijcker D, Calders P. Impact of Endurance Exercise Training in the Fasted State on Muscle Biochemistry and Metabolism in Healthy Subjects: Can These Effects be of Particular Clinical Benefit to Type 2 Diabetes Mellitus and Insulin-Resistant Patients?. Sports Med. 2017 Mar;47(3):415-428. doi: 10.1007/s40279-016-0594-x. Review. PubMed PMID: 27459862.

[266]Gjedsted J, Gormsen LC, Nielsen S, Schmitz O, Djurhuus CB, Keiding S, Ørskov H, Tønnesen E, Møller N. Effects of a 3-day fast on regional lipid and glucose metabolism in human skeletal muscle and adipose tissue. Acta Physiol (Oxf). 2007 Nov;191(3):205-16. doi: 10.1111/j.1748-1716.2007.01740.x. Epub 2007 Sep 3. PubMed PMID: 17784905.

[267]Bagherniya M, Butler AE, Barreto GE, Sahebkar A. The effect of fasting or calorie restriction on autophagy induction: A review of the literature. Ageing Res Rev. 2018 Nov;47:183-197. doi: 10.1016/j.arr.2018.08.004. Epub 2018 Aug 30. Review. PubMed PMID: 30172870.

[268]Yang JS, Lu CC, Kuo SC, Hsu YM, Tsai SC, Chen SY, Chen YT, Lin YJ, Huang YC, Chen CJ, Lin WD, Liao WL, Lin WY, Liu YH, Sheu JC, Tsai FJ. Autophagy and its link to type II diabetes mellitus. Biomedicine (Taipei). 2017 Jun;7(2):8. doi: 10.1051/bmdcn/2017070201. Epub 2017 Jun 14. PubMed PMID: 28612706; PubMed Central PMCID: PMC5479440.

[269]Mancini A, Vitucci D, Randers MB, Schmidt JF, Hagman M, Andersen TR, Imperlini E, Mandola A, Orrù S, Krustrup P, Buono P. Lifelong Football Training: Effects on Autophagy and Healthy Longevity Promotion. Front Physiol. 2019;10:132. doi: 10.3389/fphys.2019.00132. eCollection 2019. PubMed PMID: 30837897; PubMed Central PMCID: PMC6390296.

[270]He C, Sumpter R Jr, Levine B. Exercise induces autophagy in peripheral tissues and in the brain. Autophagy. 2012 Oct;8(10):1548-51. doi: 10.4161/auto.21327. Epub 2012 Aug 15. PubMed PMID: 22892563; PubMed Central PMCID: PMC3463459.

[271]Schwalm C, Jamart C, Benoit N, Naslain D, Prémont C, Prévet J, Van Thienen R, Deldicque L, Francaux M. Activation of autophagy in human skeletal muscle is dependent on exercise intensity and AMPK activation. FASEB J. 2015 Aug;29(8):3515-26. doi: 10.1096/fj.14-267187. Epub 2015 May 8. PubMed PMID: 25957282.

[272]Ho KY, Veldhuis JD, Johnson ML, Furlanetto R, Evans WS, Alberti KG, Thorner MO. Fasting enhances growth hormone secretion and amplifies the complex rhythms of growth hormone secretion in man. J Clin Invest. 1988 Apr;81(4):968-75. doi: 10.1172/JCI113450. PubMed PMID: 3127426; PubMed Central PMCID: PMC329619.

[273]Besson A, Salemi S, Gallati S, Jenal A, Horn R, Mullis PS, Mullis PE. Reduced longevity in untreated patients with isolated growth hormone deficiency. J Clin Endocrinol Metab. 2003 Aug;88(8):3664-7. doi: 10.1210/jc.2002-021938. PubMed PMID: 12915652.

[274]Stannard SR, Buckley AJ, Edge JA, Thompson MW. Adaptations to skeletal muscle with endurance exercise training in the acutely fed versus overnight-fasted state. J Sci Med Sport. 2010 Jul;13(4):465-9. doi: 10.1016/j.jsams.2010.03.002. Epub 2010 May 7. PubMed PMID: 20452283.

[275]Horowitz JF, Mora-Rodriguez R, Byerley LO, Coyle EF. Lipolytic suppression following carbohydrate ingestion limits fat oxidation during exercise. Am J Physiol. 1997 Oct;273(4):E768-75. doi: 10.1152/ajpendo.1997.273.4.E768. PubMed PMID: 9357807.

[276]Meijssen S, Cabezas MC, Ballieux CG, Derksen RJ, Bilecen S, Erkelens DW. Insulin mediated inhibition of hormone sensitive lipase activity in vivo in relation to endogenous catecholamines in healthy subjects. J Clin Endocrinol Metab. 2001 Sep;86(9):4193-7. doi: 10.1210/jcem.86.9.7794. PubMed PMID: 11549649.

[277]Patel JN, Coppack SW, Goldstein DS, Miles JM, Eisenhofer G. Norepinephrine spillover from human adipose tissue before and after a 72-hour fast. J Clin Endocrinol Metab. 2002 Jul;87(7):3373-7. doi: 10.1210/jcem.87.7.8695. PubMed PMID: 12107252.

[278]Hallböök T, Ji S, Maudsley S, Martin B. The effects of the ketogenic diet on behavior and cognition. Epilepsy Res. 2012 Jul;100(3):304-9. doi: 10.1016/j.eplepsyres.2011.04.017. Epub 2011 Aug 27. Review. PubMed PMID: 21872440; PubMed Central PMCID: PMC4112040.

How to Fight Cravings Naturally

[279]Müller TD, Nogueiras R, Andermann ML, Andrews ZB, Anker SD, Argente J, Batterham RL, Benoit SC, Bowers CY, Broglio F, Casanueva FF, D'Alessio D, Depoortere I, Geliebter A, Ghigo E, Cole PA, Cowley M, Cummings DE, Dagher A, Diano S, Dickson SL, Diéguez C, Granata R, Grill HJ, Grove K, Habegger KM, Heppner K, Heiman ML, Holsen L, Holst B, Inui A, Jansson JO, Kirchner H, Korbonits M, Laferrère B, LeRoux CW, Lopez M, Morin S, Nakazato M, Nass R, Perez-Tilve D, Pfluger PT, Schwartz TW, Seeley RJ, Sleeman M, Sun Y, Sussel L, Tong J, Thorner MO, van der Lely AJ, van der Ploeg LH, Zigman JM, Kojima M, Kangawa K, Smith RG, Horvath T, Tschöp MH. Ghrelin. Mol Metab. 2015 Jun;4(6):437-60. doi: 10.1016/j.molmet.2015.03.005. eCollection 2015 Jun. Review. PubMed PMID: 26042199; PubMed Central PMCID: PMC4443295.

[280]Blom WA, Lluch A, Stafleu A, Vinoy S, Holst JJ, Schaafsma G, Hendriks HF. Effect of a high-protein breakfast on the postprandial ghrelin response. Am J Clin Nutr. 2006 Feb;83(2):211-20. doi: 10.1093/ajcn/83.2.211. PubMed PMID: 16469977.

[281]White BD, He B, Dean RG, Martin RJ. Low protein diets increase neuropeptide Y gene expression in the basomedial hypothalamus of rats. J Nutr. 1994 Aug;124(8):1152-60. doi: 10.1093/jn/124.8.1152. PubMed PMID: 8064364.

282Beck B. Neuropeptide Y in normal eating and in genetic and dietary-induced obesity. Philos Trans R Soc Lond B Biol Sci. 2006 Jul 29;361(1471):1159-85. doi: 10.1098/rstb.2006.1855. Review. PubMed PMID: 16874931; PubMed Central PMCID: PMC1642692.

283Parra D, Ramel A, Bandarra N, Kiely M, Martínez JA, Thorsdottir I. A diet rich in long chain omega-3 fatty acids modulates satiety in overweight and obese volunteers during weight loss. Appetite. 2008 Nov;51(3):676-80. doi: 10.1016/j.appet.2008.06.003. Epub 2008 Jun 14. PubMed PMID: 18602429.

284Teff KL, Elliott SS, Tschöp M, Kieffer TJ, Rader D, Heiman M, Townsend RR, Keim NL, D'Alessio D, Havel PJ. Dietary fructose reduces circulating insulin and leptin, attenuates postprandial suppression of ghrelin, and increases triglycerides in women. J Clin Endocrinol Metab. 2004 Jun;89(6):2963-72. doi: 10.1210/jc.2003-031855. PubMed PMID: 15181085.

285Lustig RH. Fructose: it's "alcohol without the buzz". Adv Nutr. 2013 Mar 1;4(2):226-35. doi: 10.3945/an.112.002998. PubMed PMID: 23493539; PubMed Central PMCID: PMC3649103.

286Shapiro A, Mu W, Roncal C, Cheng KY, Johnson RJ, Scarpace PJ. Fructose-induced leptin resistance exacerbates weight gain in response to subsequent high-fat feeding. Am J Physiol Regul Integr Comp Physiol. 2008 Nov;295(5):R1370-5. doi: 10.1152/ajpregu.00195.2008. Epub 2008 Aug 13. PubMed PMID: 18703413; PubMed Central PMCID: PMC2584858.

287Shapiro A, Mu W, Roncal C, Cheng KY, Johnson RJ, Scarpace PJ. Fructose-induced leptin resistance exacerbates weight gain in response to subsequent high-fat feeding. Am J Physiol Regul Integr Comp Physiol. 2008 Nov;295(5):R1370-5. doi: 10.1152/ajpregu.00195.2008. Epub 2008 Aug 13. PubMed PMID: 18703413; PubMed Central PMCID: PMC2584858.

[288]Lomenick JP, Melguizo MS, Mitchell SL, Summar ML, Anderson JW. Effects of meals high in carbohydrate, protein, and fat on ghrelin and peptide YY secretion in prepubertal children. J Clin Endocrinol Metab. 2009 Nov;94(11):4463-71. doi: 10.1210/jc.2009-0949. Epub 2009 Oct 9. PubMed PMID: 19820013; PubMed Central PMCID: PMC2775646.

[289]Buyken AE, Goletzke J, Joslowski G, Felbick A, Cheng G, Herder C, Brand-Miller JC. Association between carbohydrate quality and inflammatory markers: systematic review of observational and interventional studies. Am J Clin Nutr. 2014 Apr;99(4):813-33. doi: 10.3945/ajcn.113.074252. Epub 2014 Feb 19. Review. PubMed PMID: 24552752.

[290]Gagnon J, Sauvé M, Zhao W, Stacey HM, Wiber SC, Bolz SS, Brubaker PL. Chronic Exposure to TNFα Impairs Secretion of Glucagon-Like Peptide-1. Endocrinology. 2015 Nov;156(11):3950-60. doi: 10.1210/en.2015-1361. Epub 2015 Aug 13. PubMed PMID: 26270730.

[291]Marchix J, Choque B, Kouba M, Fautrel A, Catheline D, Legrand P. Excessive dietary linoleic acid induces proinflammatory markers in rats. J Nutr Biochem. 2015 Dec;26(12):1434-41. doi: 10.1016/j.jnutbio.2015.07.010. Epub 2015 Jul 30. PubMed PMID: 26337666.

[292]Bodnaruc AM, Prud'homme D, Blanchet R, Giroux I. Nutritional modulation of endogenous glucagon-like peptide-1 secretion: a review. Nutr Metab (Lond). 2016;13:92. doi: 10.1186/s12986-016-0153-3. eCollection 2016. Review. PubMed PMID: 27990172; PubMed Central PMCID: PMC5148911.

[293]Dockray GJ. Cholecystokinin. Curr Opin Endocrinol Diabetes Obes. 2012 Feb;19(1):8-12. doi: 10.1097/MED.0b013e32834eb77d. Review. PubMed PMID: 22157397.

[294]Dirlewanger M, di Vetta V, Guenat E, Battilana P, Seematter G, Schneiter P, Jéquier E, Tappy L. Effects of short-term carbohydrate or fat overfeeding on energy expenditure and plasma leptin concentrations in healthy female subjects. Int J Obes Relat Metab Disord. 2000 Nov;24(11):1413-8. doi: 10.1038/sj.ijo.0801395. PubMed PMID: 11126336.

[295]Pironi L, Stanghellini V, Miglioli M, Corinaldesi R, De Giorgio R, Ruggeri E, Tosetti C, Poggioli G, Morselli Labate AM, Monetti N. Fat-induced ileal brake in humans: a dose-dependent phenomenon correlated to the plasma levels of peptide YY. Gastroenterology. 1993 Sep;105(3):733-9. doi: 10.1016/0016-5085(93)90890-o. PubMed PMID: 8359644.

[296]Chungchunlam SM, Henare SJ, Ganesh S, Moughan PJ. Dietary whey protein influences plasma satiety-related hormones and plasma amino acids in normal-weight adult women. Eur J Clin Nutr. 2015 Feb;69(2):179-86. doi: 10.1038/ejcn.2014.266. Epub 2015 Jan 7. PubMed PMID: 25563737.

[297]Gillespie AL, Calderwood D, Hobson L, Green BD. Whey proteins have beneficial effects on intestinal enteroendocrine cells stimulating cell growth and increasing the production and secretion of incretin hormones. Food Chem. 2015 Dec 15;189:120-8. doi: 10.1016/j.foodchem.2015.02.022. Epub 2015 Feb 18. PubMed PMID: 26190610.

[298]Rubio IG, Castro G, Zanini AC, Medeiros-Neto G. Oral ingestion of a hydrolyzed gelatin meal in subjects with normal weight and in obese patients: Postprandial effect on circulating gut peptides, glucose and insulin. Eat Weight Disord. 2008 Mar;13(1):48-53. doi: 10.1007/BF03327784. PubMed PMID: 18319637.

[299]Lomenick JP, Melguizo MS, Mitchell SL, Summar ML, Anderson JW. Effects of meals high in carbohydrate, protein, and fat on ghrelin and peptide YY secretion in prepubertal children. J Clin Endocrinol Metab. 2009 Nov;94(11):4463-71. doi: 10.1210/jc.2009-0949. Epub 2009 Oct 9. PubMed PMID: 19820013; PubMed Central PMCID: PMC2775646.

[300]Spiegel K, Leproult R, L'hermite-Balériaux M, Copinschi G, Penev PD, Van Cauter E. Leptin levels are dependent on sleep duration: relationships with sympathovagal balance, carbohydrate regulation, cortisol, and thyrotropin. J Clin Endocrinol Metab. 2004 Nov;89(11):5762-71. doi: 10.1210/jc.2004-1003. PubMed PMID: 15531540.

[301]Mosavat M, Mirsanjari M, Arabiat D, Smyth A, Whitehead L. The Role of Sleep Curtailment on Leptin Levels in Obesity and Diabetes Mellitus. Obes Facts. 2021;14(2):214-221. doi: 10.1159/000514095. Epub 2021 Mar 23. Review. PubMed PMID: 33756469; PubMed Central PMCID: PMC8138234.

[302]Cooper CB, Neufeld EV, Dolezal BA, Martin JL. Sleep deprivation and obesity in adults: a brief narrative review. BMJ Open Sport Exerc Med. 2018;4(1):e000392. doi: 10.1136/bmjsem-2018-000392. eCollection 2018. PubMed PMID: 30364557; PubMed Central PMCID: PMC6196958.

[303]Lin J, Jiang Y, Wang G, Meng M, Zhu Q, Mei H, Liu S, Jiang F. Associations of short sleep duration with appetite-regulating hormones and adipokines: A systematic review and meta-analysis. Obes Rev. 2020 Nov;21(11):e13051. doi: 10.1111/obr.13051. Epub 2020 Jun 15. Review. PubMed PMID: 32537891.

[304]Cooper CB, Neufeld EV, Dolezal BA, Martin JL. Sleep deprivation and obesity in adults: a brief narrative review. BMJ Open Sport Exerc Med. 2018;4(1):e000392. doi: 10.1136/bmjsem-2018-000392. eCollection 2018. PubMed PMID: 30364557; PubMed Central PMCID: PMC6196958.

[305]Kang S, Kim KB, Shin KO. Exercise training improves leptin sensitivity in peripheral tissue of obese rats. Biochem Biophys Res Commun. 2013 Jun 7;435(3):454-9. doi: 10.1016/j.bbrc.2013.05.007. Epub 2013 May 11. PubMed PMID: 23669042.

[306]Jones TE, Basilio JL, Brophy PM, McCammon MR, Hickner RC. Long-term exercise training in overweight adolescents improves plasma peptide YY and resistin. Obesity (Silver Spring). 2009 Jun;17(6):1189-95. doi: 10.1038/oby.2009.11. Epub 2009 Feb 26. PubMed PMID: 19247279; PubMed Central PMCID: PMC3845441.

[307]Zouhal H, Sellami M, Saeidi A, Slimani M, Abbassi-Daloii A, Khodamoradi A, El Hage R, Hackney AC, Ben Abderrahman A. Effect of physical exercise and training on gastrointestinal hormones in populations with different weight statuses. Nutr Rev. 2019 Jul 1;77(7):455-477. doi: 10.1093/nutrit/nuz005. Review. PubMed PMID: 31125091.

[308]Khajehnasiri N, Khazali H, Sheikhzadeh F, Ghowsi M. One-month of high-intensity exercise did not change the food intake and the hypothalamic arcuate nucleus proopiomelanocortin and neuropeptide Y expression levels in male Wistar rats. Endocr Regul. 2019 Jan 1;53(1):8-13. doi: 10.2478/enr-2019-0002. PubMed PMID: 31517616.

[309]Benite-Ribeiro SA, Putt DA, Santos JM. The effect of physical exercise on orexigenic and anorexigenic peptides and its role on long-term feeding control. Med Hypotheses. 2016 Aug;93:30-3. doi: 10.1016/j.mehy.2016.05.005. Epub 2016 May 11. PubMed PMID: 27372853.

[310]Melanson EL, Keadle SK, Donnelly JE, Braun B, King NA. Resistance to exercise-induced weight loss: compensatory behavioral adaptations. Med Sci Sports Exerc. 2013 Aug;45(8):1600-9. doi: 10.1249/MSS.0b013e31828ba942. Review. PubMed PMID: 23470300; PubMed Central PMCID: PMC3696411.

[311]Shapiro A, Mu W, Roncal C, Cheng KY, Johnson RJ, Scarpace PJ. Fructose-induced leptin resistance exacerbates weight gain in response to subsequent high-fat feeding. Am J Physiol Regul Integr Comp Physiol. 2008 Nov;295(5):R1370-5. doi: 10.1152/ajpregu.00195.2008. Epub 2008 Aug 13. PubMed PMID: 18703413; PubMed Central PMCID: PMC2584858.

[312]Deemer SE, Plaisance EP, Martins C. Impact of ketosis on appetite regulation-a review. Nutr Res. 2020 May;77:1-11. doi: 10.1016/j.nutres.2020.02.010. Epub 2020 Feb 20. Review. PubMed PMID: 32193016.

[313]Essah PA, Levy JR, Sistrun SN, Kelly SM, Nestler JE. Effect of macronutrient composition on postprandial peptide YY levels. J Clin Endocrinol Metab. 2007 Oct;92(10):4052-5. doi: 10.1210/jc.2006-2273. Epub 2007 Aug 28. PubMed PMID: 17726080.

[314]Michalsen A, Schlegel F, Rodenbeck A, Lüdtke R, Huether G, Teschler H, Dobos GJ. Effects of short-term modified fasting on sleep patterns and daytime vigilance in non-obese subjects: results of a pilot study. Ann Nutr Metab. 2003;47(5):194-200. doi: 10.1159/000070485. PubMed PMID: 12748412.

Diet for a Healthy Cycle

[315]Fathizadeh N, Ebrahimi E, Valiani M, Tavakoli N, Yar MH. Evaluating the effect of magnesium and magnesium plus vitamin B6 supplement on the severity of premenstrual syndrome. Iran J Nurs Midwifery Res. 2010 Dec;15(Suppl 1):401-5. PubMed PMID: 22069417; PubMed Central PMCID: PMC3208934.

[316]Zafari M, Behmanesh F, Agha Mohammadi A. Comparison of the effect of fish oil and ibuprofen on treatment of severe pain in primary dysmenorrhea. Caspian J Intern Med. 2011 Summer;2(3):279-82. PubMed PMID: 24049587; PubMed Central PMCID: PMC3770499.

[317]Weinberg ED. The hazards of iron loading. Metallomics. 2010 Nov;2(11):732-40. doi: 10.1039/c0mt00023j. Epub 2010 Sep 24. Review. PubMed PMID: 21072364.

[318]The Self NutritionData method and system [Internet]. New York: Condé Nast; c2018 [cited 2021 Jan 29]. Available from: https://nutritiondata.self.com/facts/finfish-and-shellfish-products/4189/2.

[319]The Self NutritionData method and system [Internet]. New York: Condé Nast; c2018 [cited 2021 Jan 29]. Available from: https://nutritiondata.self.com/facts/finfish-and-shellfish-products/4102/2.

[320]The Self NutritionData method and system [Internet]. New York: Condé Nast; c2018 [cited 2021 Jan 29]. Available from: https://nutritiondata.self.com/facts/poultry-products/7211/2.

[321]The Self NutritionData method and system [Internet]. New York: Condé Nast; c2018 [cited 2021 Jan 29]. Available from: https://nutritiondata.self.com/facts/beef-products/3689/2.

[322]The Self NutritionData method and system [Internet]. New York: Condé Nast; c2018 [cited 2021 Jan 29]. Available from: https://nutritiondata.self.com/facts/nut-and-seed-products/3138/2.

[323]Delgado BJ, Lopez-Ojeda W. Estrogen. 2022 Jan;. PubMed PMID: 30855848.

[324]Shors TJ, Leuner B. Estrogen-mediated effects on depression and memory formation in females. J Affect Disord. 2003 Mar;74(1):85-96. doi: 10.1016/s0165-0327(02)00428-7. PubMed PMID: 12646301; PubMed Central PMCID: PMC3374589.

[325]Michnovicz JJ, Bradlow HL. Altered estrogen metabolism and excretion in humans following consumption of indole-3-carbinol. Nutr Cancer. 1991;16(1):59-66. doi: 10.1080/01635589109514141. PubMed PMID: 1656396.

[326]Rose DP, Goldman M, Connolly JM, Strong LE. High-fiber diet reduces serum estrogen concentrations in premenopausal women. Am J Clin Nutr. 1991 Sep;54(3):520-5. doi: 10.1093/ajcn/54.3.520. PubMed PMID: 1652197.

[327]Wang LQ. Mammalian phytoestrogens: enterodiol and enterolactone. J Chromatogr B Analyt Technol Biomed Life Sci. 2002 Sep 25;777(1-2):289-309. doi: 10.1016/s1570-0232(02)00281-7. Review. PubMed PMID: 12270221.

[328]Kwan I, Onwude JL. Premenstrual syndrome. BMJ Clin Evid. 2015 Aug 25;2015. Review. PubMed PMID: 26303988; PubMed Central PMCID: PMC4548199.

[329]Perry B, Wang Y. Appetite regulation and weight control: the role of gut hormones. Nutr Diabetes. 2012 Jan 16;2:e26. doi: 10.1038/nutd.2011.21. PubMed PMID: 23154682; PubMed Central PMCID: PMC3302146.

[330]Krishnan S, Tryon RR, Horn WF, Welch L, Keim NL. Estradiol, SHBG and leptin interplay with food craving and intake across the menstrual cycle. Physiol Behav. 2016 Oct 15;165:304-12. doi: 10.1016/j.physbeh.2016.08.010. Epub 2016 Aug 12. PubMed PMID: 27527001.

[331]Fathizadeh N, Ebrahimi E, Valiani M, Tavakoli N, Yar MH. Evaluating the effect of magnesium and magnesium plus vitamin B6 supplement on the severity of premenstrual syndrome. Iran J Nurs Midwifery Res. 2010 Dec;15(Suppl 1):401-5. PubMed PMID: 22069417; PubMed Central PMCID: PMC3208934.

[332]Shobeiri F, Oshvandi K, Nazari M. Clinical effectiveness of vitamin E and vitamin B6 for improving pain severity in cyclic mastalgia. Iran J Nurs Midwifery Res. 2015 Nov-Dec;20(6):723-7. doi: 10.4103/1735-9066.170003. PubMed PMID: 26793260; PubMed Central PMCID: PMC4700694.

[333]The Self NutritionData method and system [Internet]. New York: Condé Nast; c2018 [cited 2021 Jan 29]. Available from: https://nutritiondata.self.com/facts/finfish-and-shellfish-products/4102/2.

[334]The Self NutritionData method and system [Internet]. New York: Condé Nast; c2018 [cited 2021 Jan 29]. Available from: https://nutritiondata.self.com/facts/dairy-and-egg-products/111/2.

[335]The Self NutritionData method and system [Internet]. New York: Condé Nast; c2018 [cited 2021 Jan 29]. Available from: https://nutritiondata.self.com/facts/poultry-products/7211/2.

[336]The Self NutritionData method and system [Internet]. New York: Condé Nast; c2018 [cited 2021 Jan 29]. Available from: https://nutritiondata.self.com/facts/beef-products/3689/2.

[337]The Self NutritionData method and system [Internet]. New York: Condé Nast; c2018 [cited 2021 Jan 29]. Available from: https://nutritiondata.self.com/facts/nut-and-seed-products/3135/2.

[338]The Self NutritionData method and system [Internet]. New York: Condé Nast; c2018 [cited 2021 Jan 29]. Available from: https://nutritiondata.self.com/facts/nut-and-seed-products/3135/2.

[339]Koshikawa N, Tatsunuma T, Furuya K, Seki K. Prostaglandins and premenstrual syndrome. Prostaglandins Leukot Essent Fatty Acids. 1992 Jan;45(1):33-6. doi: 10.1016/0952-3278(92)90099-5. PubMed PMID: 1546064.

[340]Facchinetti F, Borella P, Sances G, Fioroni L, Nappi RE, Genazzani AR. Oral magnesium successfully relieves premenstrual mood changes. Obstet Gynecol. 1991 Aug;78(2):177-81. PubMed PMID: 2067759.

[341]Fathizadeh N, Ebrahimi E, Valiani M, Tavakoli N, Yar MH. Evaluating the effect of magnesium and magnesium plus vitamin B6 supplement on the severity of premenstrual syndrome. Iran J Nurs Midwifery Res. 2010 Dec;15(Suppl 1):401-5. PubMed PMID: 22069417; PubMed Central PMCID: PMC3208934.

[342]The Self NutritionData method and system [Internet]. New York: Condé Nast; c2018 [cited 2021 Jan 29]. Available from: https://nutritiondata.self.com/facts/finfish-and-shellfish-products/4189/2.

[343]The Self NutritionData method and system [Internet]. New York: Condé Nast; c2018 [cited 2021 Jan 29]. Available from: https://nutritiondata.self.com/facts/finfish-and-shellfish-products/4063/2.

[344]The Self NutritionData method and system [Internet]. New York: Condé Nast; c2018 [cited 2021 Jan 29]. Available from: https://nutritiondata.self.com/facts/finfish-and-shellfish-products/4102/2.

[345]The Self NutritionData method and system [Internet]. New York: Condé Nast; c2018 [cited 2021 Jan 29]. Available from: https://nutritiondata.self.com/facts/custom/2277624/0.

[346]The Self NutritionData method and system [Internet]. New York: Condé Nast; c2018 [cited 2021 Jan 29]. Available from:

https://nutritiondata.self.com/facts/nut-and-seed-products/3085/2.

347The Self NutritionData method and system [Internet]. New York: Condé Nast; c2018 [cited 2021 Jan 29]. Available from: https://nutritiondata.self.com/facts/nut-and-seed-products/3135/2.

348The Self NutritionData method and system [Internet]. New York: Condé Nast; c2018 [cited 2021 Jan 29]. Available from: https://nutritiondata.self.com/facts/nut-and-seed-products/3138/2.

349Zafari M, Behmanesh F, Agha Mohammadi A. Comparison of the effect of fish oil and ibuprofen on treatment of severe pain in primary dysmenorrhea. Caspian J Intern Med. 2011 Summer;2(3):279-82. PubMed PMID: 24049587; PubMed Central PMCID: PMC3770499.

350Fathizadeh N, Ebrahimi E, Valiani M, Tavakoli N, Yar MH. Evaluating the effect of magnesium and magnesium plus vitamin B6 supplement on the severity of premenstrual syndrome. Iran J Nurs Midwifery Res. 2010 Dec;15(Suppl 1):401-5. PubMed PMID: 22069417; PubMed Central PMCID: PMC3208934.

351Shobeiri F, Oshvandi K, Nazari M. Clinical effectiveness of vitamin E and vitamin B6 for improving pain severity in cyclic mastalgia. Iran J Nurs Midwifery Res. 2015 Nov-Dec;20(6):723-7. doi: 10.4103/1735-9066.170003. PubMed PMID: 26793260; PubMed Central PMCID: PMC4700694.

352The Self NutritionData method and system [Internet]. New York: Condé Nast; c2018 [cited 2021 Jan 29]. Available from: https://nutritiondata.self.com/facts/custom/2277624/0.

353Food Database GmbH [Internet]. Bremen; c2021 [cited 2021 Jan 29]. Available from: https://fddb.info/db/de/lebensmittel/diverse_schokolade_72prozent/index.html.

[354]Gold EB, Wells C, Rasor MO. The Association of Inflammation with Premenstrual Symptoms. J Womens Health (Larchmt). 2016 Sep;25(9):865-74. doi: 10.1089/jwh.2015.5529. Epub 2016 May 2. PubMed PMID: 27135720; PubMed Central PMCID: PMC5311461.

[355]Teff KL, Elliott SS, Tschöp M, Kieffer TJ, Rader D, Heiman M, Townsend RR, Keim NL, D'Alessio D, Havel PJ. Dietary fructose reduces circulating insulin and leptin, attenuates postprandial suppression of ghrelin, and increases triglycerides in women. J Clin Endocrinol Metab. 2004 Jun;89(6):2963-72. doi: 10.1210/jc.2003-031855. PubMed PMID: 15181085.

[356]Rossignol AM, Bonnlander H. Prevalence and severity of the premenstrual syndrome. Effects of foods and beverages that are sweet or high in sugar content. J Reprod Med. 1991 Feb;36(2):131-6. PubMed PMID: 2010896.

[357]Buyken AE, Goletzke J, Joslowski G, Felbick A, Cheng G, Herder C, Brand-Miller JC. Association between carbohydrate quality and inflammatory markers: systematic review of observational and interventional studies. Am J Clin Nutr. 2014 Apr;99(4):813-33. doi: 10.3945/ajcn.113.074252. Epub 2014 Feb 19. Review. PubMed PMID: 24552752.

[358]Marchix J, Choque B, Kouba M, Fautrel A, Catheline D, Legrand P. Excessive dietary linoleic acid induces proinflammatory markers in rats. J Nutr Biochem. 2015 Dec;26(12):1434-41. doi: 10.1016/j.jnutbio.2015.07.010. Epub 2015 Jul 30. PubMed PMID: 26337666.

[359]Ulven SM, Kirkhus B, Lamglait A, Basu S, Elind E, Haider T, Berge K, Vik H, Pedersen JI. Metabolic effects of krill oil are essentially similar to those of fish oil but at lower dose of EPA and DHA, in healthy volunteers. Lipids. 2011 Jan;46(1):37-46. doi: 10.1007/s11745-010-3490-4. Epub 2010 Nov 2. PubMed PMID: 21042875; PubMed Central PMCID: PMC3024511.

[360]Zafari M, Behmanesh F, Agha Mohammadi A. Comparison of the effect of fish oil and ibuprofen on treatment of severe pain in primary dysmenorrhea. Caspian J Intern Med. 2011 Summer;2(3):279-82. PubMed PMID: 24049587; PubMed Central PMCID: PMC3770499.

[361]Fathizadeh N, Ebrahimi E, Valiani M, Tavakoli N, Yar MH. Evaluating the effect of magnesium and magnesium plus vitamin B6 supplement on the severity of premenstrual syndrome. Iran J Nurs Midwifery Res. 2010 Dec;15(Suppl 1):401-5. PubMed PMID: 22069417; PubMed Central PMCID: PMC3208934.

[362]Shobeiri F, Oshvandi K, Nazari M. Clinical effectiveness of vitamin E and vitamin B6 for improving pain severity in cyclic mastalgia. Iran J Nurs Midwifery Res. 2015 Nov-Dec;20(6):723-7. doi: 10.4103/1735-9066.170003. PubMed PMID: 26793260; PubMed Central PMCID: PMC4700694.

How to Break a Weight Loss Plateau

[363]Partridge D, Lloyd KA, Rhodes JM, Walker AW, Johnstone AM, Campbell BJ. Food additives: Assessing the impact of exposure to permitted emulsifiers on bowel and metabolic health – introducing the FADiets study. Nutr Bull. 2019 Dec;44(4):329-349. doi: 10.1111/nbu.12408. Epub 2019 Nov 25. PubMed PMID: 31866761; PubMed Central PMCID: PMC6899614.

[364]Hrncirova L, Hudcovic T, Sukova E, Machova V, Trckova E, Krejsek J, Hrncir T. Human gut microbes are susceptible to antimicrobial food additives in vitro. Folia Microbiol (Praha). 2019 Jul;64(4):497-508. doi: 10.1007/s12223-018-00674-z. Epub 2019 Jan 17. PubMed PMID: 30656592.

[365]Austin J, Marks D. Hormonal regulators of appetite. Int J Pediatr Endocrinol. 2009;2009:141753. doi: 10.1155/2009/141753. Epub 2008 Dec 3. PubMed PMID: 19946401; PubMed Central PMCID: PMC2777281.

[366]Teff KL, Elliott SS, Tschöp M, Kieffer TJ, Rader D, Heiman M, Townsend RR, Keim NL, D'Alessio D, Havel PJ. Dietary fructose reduces circulating insulin and leptin, attenuates postprandial suppression of ghrelin, and increases triglycerides in women. J Clin Endocrinol Metab. 2004 Jun;89(6):2963-72. doi: 10.1210/jc.2003-031855. PubMed PMID: 15181085.

[367]Wien M, Haddad E, Oda K, Sabaté J. A randomized 3×3 crossover study to evaluate the effect of Hass avocado intake on post-ingestive satiety, glucose and insulin levels, and subsequent energy intake in overweight adults. Nutr J. 2013 Nov 27;12:155. doi: 10.1186/1475-2891-12-155. PubMed PMID: 24279738; PubMed Central PMCID: PMC4222592.

[368]Nuttall FQ, Gannon MC. Plasma glucose and insulin response to macronutrients in nondiabetic and NIDDM subjects. Diabetes Care. 1991 Sep;14(9):824-38. doi: 10.2337/diacare.14.9.824. Review. PubMed PMID: 1959475.

[369]Macedo ML, Oliveira CF, Oliveira CT. Insecticidal activity of plant lectins and potential application in crop protection. Molecules. 2015 Jan 27;20(2):2014-33. doi: 10.3390/molecules20022014. Review. PubMed PMID: 25633332; PubMed Central PMCID: PMC6272522.

[370]Freed DL. Do dietary lectins cause disease?. BMJ. 1999 Apr 17;318(7190):1023-4. doi: 10.1136/bmj.318.7190.1023. PubMed PMID: 10205084; PubMed Central PMCID: PMC1115436.

[371]Shechter Y. Bound lectins that mimic insulin produce persistent insulin-like activities. Endocrinology. 1983 Dec;113(6):1921-6. doi: 10.1210/endo-113-6-1921. PubMed PMID: 6357762.

[372]Dalla Pellegrina C, Perbellini O, Scupoli MT, Tomelleri C, Zanetti C, Zoccatelli G, Fusi M, Peruffo A, Rizzi C, Chignola R. Effects of wheat germ agglutinin on human gastrointestinal epithelium: insights from an experimental model of immune/epithelial cell interaction. Toxicol Appl Pharmacol. 2009 Jun 1;237(2):146-53. doi: 10.1016/j.taap.2009.03.012. Epub 2009 Mar 28. PubMed PMID: 19332085.

373Owen OE, Cahill GF Jr. Metabolic effects of exogenous glu-cocorticoids in fasted man. J Clin Invest. 1973 Oct;52(10):2596-605. doi: 10.1172/JCI107452. PubMed PMID: 4729053; PubMed Central PMCID: PMC302520.

374Rizza RA, Mandarino LJ, Gerich JE. Cortisol-induced insulin resistance in man: impaired suppression of glucose production and stimulation of glucose utilization due to a postreceptor de-tect of insulin action. J Clin Endocrinol Metab. 1982 Jan;54(1):131-8. doi: 10.1210/jcem-54-1-131. PubMed PMID: 7033265.

375Ayachi SE, Paulmyer-Lacroix O, Verdier M, Alessi MC, Dutour A, Grino M. 11beta-Hydroxysteroid dehydrogenase type 1-dri-ven cortisone reactivation regulates plasminogen activator in-hibitor type 1 in adipose tissue of obese women. J Thromb Ha-emost. 2006 Mar;4(3):621-7. doi: 10.1111/j.1538-7836.2006.01811.x. PubMed PMID: 16460444.

376Cappuccio FP, Taggart FM, Kandala NB, Currie A, Peile E, Stranges S, Miller MA. Meta-analysis of short sleep duration and obesity in children and adults. Sleep. 2008 May;31(5):619-26. doi: 10.1093/sleep/31.5.619. PubMed PMID: 18517032; PubMed Central PMCID: PMC2398753.

377Taheri S, Lin L, Austin D, Young T, Mignot E. Short sleep du-ration is associated with reduced leptin, elevated ghrelin, and increased body mass index. PLoS Med. 2004 Dec;1(3):e62. doi: 10.1371/journal.pmed.0010062. Epub 2004 Dec 7. PubMed PMID: 15602591; PubMed Central PMCID: PMC535701.

378Hackney AC. Stress and the neuroendocrine system: the role of exercise as a stressor and modifier of stress. Expert Rev En-docrinol Metab. 2006 Nov 1;1(6):783-792. doi: 10.1586/17446651.1.6.783. PubMed PMID: 20948580; Pub-Med Central PMCID: PMC2953272.

379Meczekalski B, Katulski K, Czyzyk A, Podfigurna-Stopa A, Maciejewska-Jeske M. Functional hypothalamic amenorrhea and its influence on women's health. J Endocrinol Invest. 2014 Nov;37(11):1049-56. doi: 10.1007/s40618-014-0169-3. Epub 2014 Sep 9. Review. PubMed PMID: 25201001; PubMed Central PMCID: PMC4207953.

380Anton SD, Martin CK, Han H, Coulon S, Cefalu WT, Geiselman P, Williamson DA. Effects of stevia, aspartame, and sucrose on food intake, satiety, and postprandial glucose and insulin levels. Appetite. 2010 Aug;55(1):37-43. doi: 10.1016/j.appet.2010.03.009. Epub 2010 Mar 18. PubMed PMID: 20303371; PubMed Central PMCID: PMC2900484.

381Jeppesen PB, Gregersen S, Poulsen CR, Hermansen K. Stevioside acts directly on pancreatic beta cells to secrete insulin: actions independent of cyclic adenosine monophosphate and adenosine triphosphate-sensitive K+-channel activity. Metabolism. 2000 Feb;49(2):208-14. doi: 10.1016/s0026-0495(00)91325-8. PubMed PMID: 10690946.

382Zhou Y, Zheng Y, Ebersole J, Huang CF. Insulin secretion stimulating effects of mogroside V and fruit extract of luo han kuo (Siraitia grosvenori Swingle) fruit extract.. Yao Xue Xue Bao. 2009 Nov;44(11):1252-7. PubMed PMID: 21351724.

383Ruiz-Ojeda FJ, Plaza-Díaz J, Sáez-Lara MJ, Gil A. Effects of Sweeteners on the Gut Microbiota: A Review of Experimental Studies and Clinical Trials. Adv Nutr. 2019 Jan 1;10(suppl_1):S31-S48. doi: 10.1093/advances/nmy037. PubMed PMID: 30721958; PubMed Central PMCID: PMC6363527.

384Yang Q. Gain weight by "going diet?" Artificial sweeteners and the neurobiology of sugar cravings: Neuroscience 2010. Yale J Biol Med. 2010 Jun;83(2):101-8. Review. PubMed PMID: 20589192; PubMed Central PMCID: PMC2892765

[385]Fowler SP, Williams K, Resendez RG, Hunt KJ, Hazuda HP, Stern MP. Fueling the obesity epidemic? Artificially sweetened beverage use and long-term weight gain. Obesity (Silver Spring). 2008 Aug;16(8):1894-900. doi: 10.1038/oby.2008.284. Epub 2008 Jun 5. PubMed PMID: 18535548.

Boost Fat Burning With Keto

[386]Nuttall FQ, Gannon MC. Plasma glucose and insulin response to macronutrients in nondiabetic and NIDDM subjects. Diabetes Care. 1991 Sep;14(9):824-38. doi: 10.2337/diacare.14.9.824. Review. PubMed PMID: 1959475.

[387]LaManna JC, Salem N, Puchowicz M, Erokwu B, Koppaka S, Flask C, Lee Z. Ketones suppress brain glucose consumption. Adv Exp Med Biol. 2009;645:301-6. doi: 10.1007/978-0-387-85998-9_45. PubMed PMID: 19227486; PubMed Central PMCID: PMC2874681.

[388]Patel JN, Coppack SW, Goldstein DS, Miles JM, Eisenhofer G. Norepinephrine spillover from human adipose tissue before and after a 72-hour fast. J Clin Endocrinol Metab. 2002 Jul;87(7):3373-7. doi: 10.1210/jcem.87.7.8695. PubMed PMID: 12107252.

30-Day Intermittent Fasting Challenge

[389]Yang Q. Gain weight by "going diet?" Artificial sweeteners and the neurobiology of sugar cravings: Neuroscience 2010. Yale J Biol Med. 2010 Jun;83(2):101-8. PMID: 20589192; PMCID: PMC2892765.

[390]Anton SD, Martin CK, Han H, Coulon S, Cefalu WT, Geiselman P, Williamson DA. Effects of stevia, aspartame, and sucrose on food intake, satiety, and postprandial glucose and insulin levels. Appetite. 2010 Aug;55(1):37-43. doi: 10.1016/j.appet.2010.03.009. Epub 2010 Mar 18. PubMed PMID: 20303371; PubMed Central PMCID: PMC2900484.

[391]Liang Y, Steinbach G, Maier V, Pfeiffer EF. The effect of artificial sweetener on insulin secretion. 1. The effect of acesulfame K on insulin secretion in the rat (studies in vivo). Horm Metab Res. 1987 Jun;19(6):233-8. doi: 10.1055/s-2007-1011788. PubMed PMID: 2887500.

[392]Pepino MY, Tiemann CD, Patterson BW, Wice BM, Klein S. Sucralose affects glycemic and hormonal responses to an oral glucose load. Diabetes Care. 2013 Sep;36(9):2530-5. doi: 10.2337/dc12-2221. Epub 2013 Apr 30. PubMed PMID: 23633524; PubMed Central PMCID: PMC3747933.

[393]Jeppesen PB, Gregersen S, Poulsen CR, Hermansen K. Stevioside acts directly on pancreatic beta cells to secrete insulin: actions independent of cyclic adenosine monophosphate and adenosine triphosphate-sensitive K+-channel activity. Metabolism. 2000 Feb;49(2):208-14. doi: 10.1016/s0026-0495(00)91325-8. PubMed PMID: 10690946.

[394]Zhou Y, Zheng Y, Ebersole J, Huang CF. Insulin secretion stimulating effects of mogroside V and fruit extract of luo han kuo (Siraitia grosvenori Swingle) fruit extract.. Yao Xue Xue Bao. 2009 Nov;44(11):1252-7. PubMed PMID: 21351724.

[395]Lenoir M, Serre F, Cantin L, Ahmed SH. Intense sweetness surpasses cocaine reward. PLoS One. 2007 Aug 1;2(8):e698. doi: 10.1371/journal.pone.0000698. PubMed PMID: 17668074; PubMed Central PMCID: PMC1931610.

[396]Teff KL, Elliott SS, Tschöp M, Kieffer TJ, Rader D, Heiman M, Townsend RR, Keim NL, D'Alessio D, Havel PJ. Dietary fructose reduces circulating insulin and leptin, attenuates postprandial suppression of ghrelin, and increases triglycerides in women. J Clin Endocrinol Metab. 2004 Jun;89(6):2963-72. doi: 10.1210/jc.2003-031855. PubMed PMID: 15181085.

[397]Ramsden CE, Zamora D, Leelarthaepin B, Majchrzak-Hong SF, Faurot KR, Suchindran CM, Ringel A, Davis JM, Hibbeln JR. Use of dietary linoleic acid for secondary prevention of coronary heart disease and death: evaluation of recovered data from the Sydney Diet Heart Study and updated meta-analysis. BMJ. 2013 Feb 4;346:e8707. doi: 10.1136/bmj.e8707. PubMed PMID: 23386268; PubMed Central PMCID: PMC4688426.

[398]Partridge D, Lloyd KA, Rhodes JM, Walker AW, Johnstone AM, Campbell BJ. Food additives: Assessing the impact of exposure to permitted emulsifiers on bowel and metabolic health – introducing the FADiets study. Nutr Bull. 2019 Dec;44(4):329-349. doi: 10.1111/nbu.12408. Epub 2019 Nov 25. PubMed PMID: 31866761; PubMed Central PMCID: PMC6899614.

[399]Hrncirova L, Hudcovic T, Sukova E, Machova V, Trckova E, Krejsek J, Hrncir T. Human gut microbes are susceptible to antimicrobial food additives in vitro. Folia Microbiol (Praha). 2019 Jul;64(4):497-508. doi: 10.1007/s12223-018-00674-z. Epub 2019 Jan 17. PubMed PMID: 30656592.

[400]Chandalia M, Garg A, Lutjohann D, von Bergmann K, Grundy SM, Brinkley LJ. Beneficial effects of high dietary fiber intake in patients with type 2 diabetes mellitus. N Engl J Med. 2000 May 11;342(19):1392-8. doi: 10.1056/NEJM200005113421903. PubMed PMID: 10805824.

[401]Carlson LE, Speca M, Patel KD, Goodey E. Mindfulness-based stress reduction in relation to quality of life, mood, symptoms of stress and levels of cortisol, dehydroepiandrosterone sulfate (DHEAS) and melatonin in breast and prostate cancer outpatients. Psychoneuroendocrinology. 2004 May;29(4):448-74. doi: 10.1016/s0306-4530(03)00054-4. PubMed PMID: 14749092.

[402]Klimes-Dougan B, Chong LS, Samikoglu A, Thai M, Amatya P, Cullen KR, Lim KO. Transcendental meditation and hypothalamic-pituitary-adrenal axis functioning: a pilot, randomized controlled trial with young adults. Stress. 2020 Jan;23(1):105-115. doi: 10.1080/10253890.2019.1656714. Epub 2019 Sep 11. PubMed PMID: 31418329.

[403]Pascoe MC, Thompson DR, Ski CF. Yoga, mindfulness-based stress reduction and stress-related physiological measures: A meta-analysis. Psychoneuroendocrinology. 2017 Dec;86:152-168. doi: 10.1016/j.psyneuen.2017.08.008. Epub 2017 Aug 30. PubMed PMID: 28963884.

[404]Reid KJ, Santostasi G, Baron KG, Wilson J, Kang J, Zee PC. Timing and intensity of light correlate with body weight in adults. PLoS One. 2014;9(4):e92251. doi: 10.1371/journal.pone.0092251. eCollection 2014. PubMed PMID: 24694994; PubMed Central PMCID: PMC3973603.

[405]Zouhal H, Saeidi A, Salhi A, Li H, Essop MF, Laher I, Rhibi F, Amani-Shalamzari S, Ben Abderrahman A. Exercise Training and Fasting: Current Insights. Open Access J Sports Med. 2020;11:1-28. doi: 10.2147/OAJSM.S224919. eCollection 2020. Review. PubMed PMID: 32021500; PubMed Central PMCID: PMC6983467.

[406]Schönfeld P, Wojtczak L. Short- and medium-chain fatty acids in energy metabolism: the cellular perspective. J Lipid Res. 2016 Jun;57(6):943-54. doi: 10.1194/jlr.R067629. Epub 2016 Apr 14. Review. PubMed PMID: 27080715; PubMed Central PMCID: PMC4878196.

[407]D C Harvey CJ, Schofield GM, Williden M, McQuillan JA. The Effect of Medium Chain Triglycerides on Time to Nutritional Ketosis and Symptoms of Keto-Induction in Healthy Adults: A Randomised Controlled Clinical Trial. J Nutr Metab. 2018;2018:2630565. doi: 10.1155/2018/2630565. eCollection 2018. PubMed PMID: 29951312; PubMed Central PMCID: PMC5987302.

[408]Acheson KJ, Zahorska-Markiewicz B, Pittet P, Anantharaman K, Jéquier E. Caffeine and coffee: their influence on metabolic rate and substrate utilization in normal weight and obese individuals. Am J Clin Nutr. 1980 May;33(5):989-97. doi: 10.1093/ajcn/33.5.989. PubMed PMID: 7369170.

[409]St-Onge MP, Ross R, Parsons WD, Jones PJ. Medium-chain triglycerides increase energy expenditure and decrease adiposity in overweight men. Obes Res. 2003 Mar;11(3):395-402. doi: 10.1038/oby.2003.53. PubMed PMID: 12634436.

[410]Marciani L, Cox EF, Pritchard SE, Major G, Hoad CL, Mellows M, Hussein MO, Costigan C, Fox M, Gowland PA, Spiller RC. Additive effects of gastric volumes and macronutrient composition on the sensation of postprandial fullness in humans. Eur J Clin Nutr. 2015 Mar;69(3):380-4. doi: 10.1038/ejcn.2014.194. Epub 2014 Sep 17. PubMed PMID: 25226819; PubMed Central PMCID: PMC4351404.

[411]McLaughlin JT, Lomax RB, Hall L, Dockray GJ, Thompson DG, Warhurst G. Fatty acids stimulate cholecystokinin secretion via an acyl chain length-specific, Ca2+-dependent mechanism in the enteroendocrine cell line STC-1. J Physiol. 1998 Nov 15;513 (Pt 1):11-8. doi: 10.1111/j.1469-7793.1998.011by.x. PubMed PMID: 9782155; PubMed Central PMCID: PMC2231256.

Conclusion

[412]Catenacci VA, Pan Z, Ostendorf D, Brannon S, Gozansky WS, Mattson MP, Martin B, MacLean PS, Melanson EL, Troy Donahoo W. A randomized pilot study comparing zero-calorie alternate-day fasting to daily caloric restriction in adults with obesity. Obesity (Silver Spring). 2016 Sep;24(9):1874-83. doi: 10.1002/oby.21581. PubMed PMID: 27569118; PubMed Central PMCID: PMC5042570.

[413]Martin B, Pearson M, Kebejian L, Golden E, Keselman A, Bender M, Carlson O, Egan J, Ladenheim B, Cadet JL, Becker KG, Wood W, Duffy K, Vinayakumar P, Maudsley S, Mattson MP. Sex-dependent metabolic, neuroendocrine, and cognitive responses to dietary energy restriction and excess. Endocrinology. 2007 Sep;148(9):4318-33. doi: 10.1210/en.2007-0161. Epub 2007 Jun 14. PubMed PMID: 17569758; PubMed Central PMCID: PMC2622430.

[414]Catenacci VA, Pan Z, Ostendorf D, Brannon S, Gozansky WS, Mattson MP, Martin B, MacLean PS, Melanson EL, Troy Donahoo W. A randomized pilot study comparing zero-calorie alternate-day fasting to daily caloric restriction in adults with obesity. Obesity (Silver Spring). 2016 Sep;24(9):1874-83. doi: 10.1002/oby.21581. PubMed PMID: 27569118; PubMed Central PMCID: PMC5042570.

[415]Lomenick JP, Melguizo MS, Mitchell SL, Summar ML, Anderson JW. Effects of meals high in carbohydrate, protein, and fat on ghrelin and peptide YY secretion in prepubertal children. J Clin Endocrinol Metab. 2009 Nov;94(11):4463-71. doi: 10.1210/jc.2009-0949. Epub 2009 Oct 9. PubMed PMID: 19820013; PubMed Central PMCID: PMC2775646.

[416]Nuttall FQ, Almokayyad RM, Gannon MC. The ghrelin and leptin responses to short-term starvation vs a carbohydrate-free diet in men with type 2 diabetes; a controlled, cross-over design study. Nutr Metab (Lond). 2016;13:47. doi: 10.1186/s12986-016-0106-x. eCollection 2016. PubMed PMID: 27453716; PubMed Central PMCID: PMC4957917.

[417]Orgel E, Mittelman SD. The links between insulin resistance, diabetes, and cancer. Curr Diab Rep. 2013 Apr;13(2):213-22. doi: 10.1007/s11892-012-0356-6. Review. PubMed PMID: 23271574; PubMed Central PMCID: PMC3595327.

About the Author

Mag. Stephan Lederer, BSc, MSc, is the author of the Intermittent Fasting Book Series and one of the fastest-growing health blogs in the world. Hence, more than one million women trust his evidence-based content annually.

As a former strategy consultant to global corporations, he knows that the food industry has also optimized its production costs enormously over the past decades.

Natural ingredients have been successively replaced with cheaper options wherever possible.

Nevertheless, the blind trust in the industrialization of food is at an all-time high.

That's why modern diseases are skyrocketing, even though people have never tried so hard to live healthily.

Stephan is convinced that it's not your fault if you haven't gotten into the physical and mental shape you and your loved ones deserve.

The truth is that food and pharma lobbies have been lecturing us for decades about what is good for us.

Because of this, the common perception of health is light years away from the scientifically proven reality.

As a result, you will not find more conflicting information in any other sector than in nutrition.

Since several multi-billion dollar industries have been built on the wrong definition of what is healthy, little will change in the future.

Therefore, he believes it is solely in our hands to regain control over our health.

With this book, you already have a clear guide that can lead you to a more confident, happier, and dynamic future.

In addition, Stephan provides carefully researched knowledge in simple terms for free at www.mentalfoodchain.com.

He aims to help you rebalance your hormones, lose weight, regain control of your health, and eventually live longer and happier.

Stephan's data-driven approach allows you to distinguish between trends and evidence. He strictly rejects mere claims and always shows the current state of research.

You can find even more about the author at www.mentalfoodchain.com/about/.

Disclaimer

The contents of this book have been checked and prepared with great care. However, the author cannot guarantee or warranty the contents' completeness, accuracy, and timeliness.

This book's content represents the author's personal experience and opinion and is only intended for informational and entertainment purposes. Therefore, no legal responsibility or guarantee for the success of the mentioned tips and advice can be assumed. The author assumes no responsibility for the non-achievement of the goals described in the book.

This book contains links to other websites. The author has no influence on the content of these websites. Therefore, the author cannot take responsibility for this content. The respective provider or operator of the pages is responsible for the content of the linked pages. Illegal contents could not be determined at the time of linking.

Contact

Intermittent Fasting 16/8 for Women

Achieve Hormone Harmony to Lose Weight Fast Without Losing Your Mind – Incl. 30-Day Fasting Challenge and Meal Plan

1. Edition

ISBN: 9798839103382

Mag. Stephan Lederer, Bakk., MSc, Sigmundstadl 20/3, AT-8020 Graz

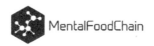

www.mentalfoodchain.com

Printed in Great Britain
by Amazon